Dental First Aid
for Families

Richard Diamond, DDS

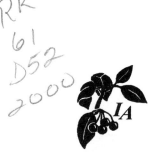

Idyll Arbor, Inc.

PO Box 720, Ravensdale, WA 98051 (425) 432-3231

Idyll Arbor, Inc. Editor: joan burlingame

Library of Congress Cataloging-in-Publication Data

```
Diamond, Richard, 1936 -
   Dental first aid for families / Richard Diamond.
      p.     cm. -- (An Idyll Arbor personal health
   book)
   ISBN 1-882883-39-X
   1. Teeth -- Care and hygiene.  2. Dental
   emergencies Popular works.
   I. Title.  II Series.
RK61.D52    1999
617.6'01 -- dc21
                                            99-40278
                                               CIP
```

Dedication

This book is dedicated to my folks without whose support, both moral and financial, I would never have been able to complete dental school. They were always there to listen to my gripes and complaints (of which there were many) and always, without questions, worked those extra hours in their small neighborhood grocery store to generate the funds necessary for my schooling. How they did it, I'll never know.

I never lacked anything. I was even able to have a car, which was an unheard of luxury for a college student attending professional school. I must admit, I did have to push the car every morning to get it started, but it was far better than walking to school.

Thank you both from the bottom of my heart.

Contents

Forward

"How can I fix it when my dentist is nowhere around?"

I don't claim to be a super-dentist. I was in general practice for thirty-five years before I retired, always in the same location. Nobody to date has tried to shoot me. At least I haven't been hit yet.

My practice was located in a blue-collar neighborhood where a dollar had to be stretched. For over three decades I tried my best, with great concern, to help accomplish that goal for my patients and I hope to accomplish that here, for you.

In 1960, I graduated from the University of California Dental School, located in San Francisco, California. After graduation, I immediately enlisted in the Air Force. My reasoning was simple. At that time, the military was still drafting professionals, so I saw no logical reason to begin a civilian practice, only to be called into the service. I spent two very rewarding, learning, enjoyable years (my residency, if you will) in the Air Force. Then I was ready for private practice.

I established my office in the town where I was raised. Initially, the nucleus of my practice was comprised of immediate family (at no charge, of course) and a number of my old high school classmates who were courageous enough to give me a try. Ultimately, I worked not only on my high school buddies, but on their children and their grandchildren, among countless others in the community. Thirty-five years flew by. To this day I don't know where the time went.

My dad owned a small neighborhood grocery store in town and he never failed to throw a couple of my business cards into each bag of groceries. I hate to admit it (and please don't tell anyone) but he also gave candy to the kids in the neighborhood.

My mom was my receptionist for about twenty years. At first I was somewhat hesitant about hiring her. Who would be the boss in the office? Would there be a power struggle? My fears were rapidly dissipated. I even got used to calling her by her first name (in the office only, mind you) and my collections were never better.

To the best of my knowledge, there are no easy-to-understand, non-technical books on basic, home dental remedies and simple, do-it-yourself repairs of dental appliances. Call it "dental first aid" if you want. This book serves as the first of its kind.

I will grant you, most of these remedies and repairs are only temporary, to buy time, but they're certainly far better than no treatment at all. Agreed?

None of these facts is a deep, dark secret. Each one is quite easy and very fundamental. The problem, as far as I can determine, is that none of this data was readily available in one concise location. Oh, there's a smattering of information here and a bit over there, but no one has condensed things into an easy to read and understandable publication. Now someone has, me.

If this book can prevent a little pain, give you a chuckle or two, impart a bit of knowledge, save some time and aggravation, along with saving you a few bucks, then I'll feel good, because I will have accomplished what I set out to do.

Chapter 1: Introduction

This book is meant to be a reference only! It is not to be used as a definitive treatment guide. If there is a dental or medical problem, always, without hesitation, contact your health care professional for definitive diagnosis and treatment.

I will attempt to make some suggestions that may at least help to minimize certain oral problems, until you can force yourself into the dental office.

I have tried to organize this book so that you can find what you need quickly. You may use this book's Table of Contents and Index to find what you want. The back cover lists what to do in the few cases of dental problems that are real, time-critical emergencies. You may also want to read some or all of the book *before* you need it. To help you pick and choose which chapters are the most important to you, I will summarize them below. Of course, I have no objections if you read the entire book in just one sitting!

Before we get to the meat of the book, I'd like to start with a brief discussion about the mouth and what happens to it at certain ages. This brief discussion can be found in Chapter 2: What's Normal. I've simply and arbitrarily created the following groupings: infants, children, teenagers, adults and seniors.

Naturally, there will almost always be overlapping. Certain conditions exist within all of the groupings. I'll try not to be repetitive and I don't intend to even come close to covering everything.

Chapter 3 deals with what we all see as the major concern of dentistry: teeth. This chapter is a mix of preventative actions and first aid associated with such problems as pain, chips, loss of some or all of a tooth, discoloration and "things" stuck between the teeth.

Chapter 4 addresses prevention and first aid for the tissue in and around the mouth. Here you will find the "whole trooth" about everything from teething, to stopping bleeding, to gum problems. (Gum care is extremely important!) And for those of you who love pizza as much as I do, I have also thrown in information on first aid for burns to the top of the mouth.

Chapter 5 looks at braces: once the rite of passage of teenagers and now a growing part of adulthood. I cover basic first aid for annoyances such as orthodontic wires digging into your cheeks or gums. I'd like also to tell you that I will cover the annoyance of the orthodontist's bill, but sorry, I don't want to go broke.

Chapter 6 covers many of the concerns about dentures, again including preventative care as well as first aid for both you and your broken, chipped, clickety-clacking-like-train-wheels-on-railroad-tracks, or poorly fitting dentures.

Chapter 7 is my chapter for "other" preventative and first aid concerns associated with your mouth and teeth including chapped lips, bad breath, jaw pain, laryngitis and grinding of teeth.

Chapter 8 gives you the information you need to be ready for dental first aid emergencies and talks about the supplies needed for preventative care. Dental first aid kits are so easy to complete and take up so little room.

I hope that this book gives you more confidence about what you can do for your family's dental first aid and preventative care needs. If I am able to give you even one night's better rest, I have succeeded!

Emergency Dentistry

There are a few situations where you really need to get to a dentist or other health care provider as soon as possible. The most important ones regarding the mouth are listed on the inside back cover.

If you experience one of these emergencies and you can't immediately reach your own dentist, the next best thing to do is to explain the problem briefly to his/her answering service. The operator should have a referral dentist available for you rather rapidly. Your dentist should have someone available who can see you without a delay.

This is one of the purposes of an answering service. When I was away from the office, on vacation, or was unavailable for any reason, my exchange always had at least two referral numbers available in case of emergency.

If a referral number is not available, call a friend or relative for their dentist's name and number. Then suggest to your dentist that s/he make referral numbers available. If s/he doesn't, find a dentist who will.

Some areas have a twenty-four hour emergency referral service. It would be a good idea to check with your local Dental Society to see if such a service is available in your area. This, of course, should be done *long before the need for such a number*. There is a place on the inside back cover to write the number so you can find it when you really need it.

Chapter 2: What's Normal?

Eruption Dates of Baby Teeth

I don't like to give specific dates as to when teeth erupt because they are only approximations, and parents have a tendency to become overly concerned if the teeth don't come in exactly on time. There is no "exactly on time." Besides, you can't do anything about improper eruption at this stage of development anyway. The infant is far too young to have any type of treatment.

After having warned you not to worry, here's the sequence of eruption and the average ages of the infant when the teeth are supposed to come in. (There's a picture on the next page.) You'll probably go ahead and worry anyway, won't you?

The first teeth to erupt (usually) are the bottom two front teeth (central incisors), at about six to ten months of age. These are closely followed by the upper two front teeth, erupting somewhere between eight and twelve months. The upper and lower side teeth (lateral incisors) that are located directly next to the front teeth come in at nine to sixteen months.

The first baby molars come in at around thirteen to nineteen months. Canine teeth (cuspids) are next, sixteen to twenty-three months. The last baby teeth to erupt are the second molars, showing themselves around twenty-three to thirty months.

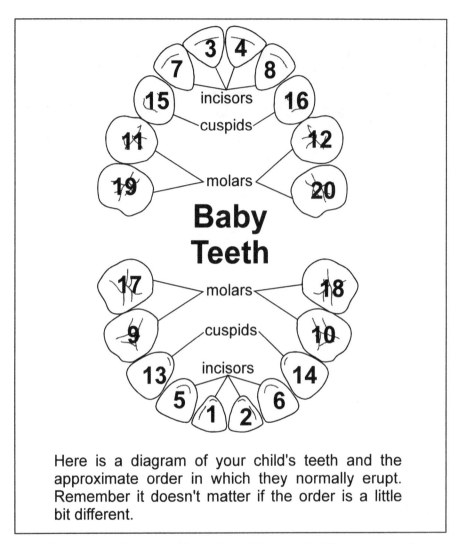

Here is a diagram of your child's teeth and the approximate order in which they normally erupt. Remember it doesn't matter if the order is a little bit different.

There you have it, for what it's worth. Twenty teeth in all: eight incisors, four canines and eight molars. The entire mouthful of baby teeth, deciduous teeth, milk teeth, primary teeth (which are all synonyms) begin erupting at about six months and the process is completed by about two or two and a half years of age.

There are, of course, conditions that are associated with certain developmental defects in which some of the tooth-buds are either improperly formed in the embryo or not formed at all. These situations are infrequent and are usually associated with other defects. It is not my intention, other than to mention them in passing, to get involved in these atypical complications.

Let's just carry this one step further with a personal note. My younger daughter has a beautiful eleven-month-old boy (the second of my three grandsons). His two lower front teeth came in at about ten months. From about seven months on, my daughter kept questioning me, "Pops, why doesn't Chase have any teeth yet? What's wrong?" I comforted my daughter as best I could, explaining to her that teeth can be somewhat tardy in erupting and it really doesn't mean much at all. Not to worry. "They will come in," I told her. I was right. End of problem? Not on your life. Immediately after they erupted, her next question to me was, "Pops, why are those two bottom teeth coming in so crooked?" I gave her a twofold answer.

First, I told her that there are many different forces at work in an infant's mouth. The initial positioning of the teeth, when they first come in, will change drastically as other teeth push their way through the gums. This, by the way, also holds true for the erupting permanent teeth.

Second, let's make an assumption. Let's assume that the teeth on my beautiful ten-month-old grandson are crooked and don't change. What can be done to correct this problem? *Absolutely nothing!* A ten month old won't take too kindly to any orthodontic treatment. Don't forget, all these baby teeth fall out. Straightening, if necessary, is primarily done on permanent teeth after they have erupted. That doesn't occur until about age twelve or thirteen. Please, don't worry now.

Spacing

Nice, straight baby teeth, with no spacing between them, are picture pretty, but beware. This could be a warning that future tooth straightening may be in the cards.

It would be preferable to see baby teeth with slight spacing between them, even as much as 1/32nd of an inch between each tooth. Permanent teeth are somewhat wider than their baby counterparts; therefore, some spacing is desirable in order to accommodate the added width. I repeat, don't concern yourself now. The only thing you can do if you encounter this potential space problem is to start saving. You'll have a good eleven or twelve years to stash the cash.

Thumb Sucking

Infants and sucking go hand in hand. They suck the breast, the bottle, the pacifier and, when the thumb is located, they latch onto it like a gourmet meal. Tremendous suction is generated and, over the years, the constant pressure can cause severe bite and jaw problems, the most common being an overbite condition (bucktooth appearance).

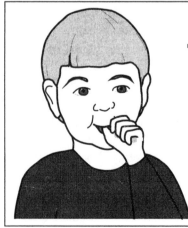

Thumbsucking

It's not horrible for your child so you might as well let it go, at least until your child is old enough for school. There isn't much you can do about it anyway.

Don't yell, don't threaten, don't bribe. It won't do any good. Anti-thumb-sucking devices aren't any more effective. Thankfully, the habit is self-limiting and usually stops by or before school age.

Brushing

Obviously, a two or three year old doesn't have the coordination (nor the desire) to brush his or her teeth properly. There are, however, a couple of things you can do to help develop the "brushing habit."

Toothpaste is very pleasant tasting to a youngster. Put the slightest amount (to taste) on a washcloth and, when you've finished brushing your own teeth (while your child watches in amazement), you can quite adequately help clean baby's teeth by rubbing them with the cloth. After a while I'll bet anything that the baby will want to try it alone. Always start or finish the session by completing the job yourself. You'll be doing the real cleaning. Baby will be playing. He or she will probably be doing it for the flavor of the paste, but it's a start in the development of a lifelong habit that many teens and adults have never quite mastered.

A number of the toy stores sell swallow-proof "baby safe" toothbrushes. I think they're terrific appliances. They are specially designed for youngsters who have not yet developed the coordination to use a conventional brush. Baby is just playing, but playing and enjoyment are precursors to learning.

Fillings

There is a common misconception that baby teeth don't have to be filled because they're going to be lost anyway.

Why subject the youngster to the discomfort and why subject yourself to the expense of fillings, if this is the case?

If the tooth involved is close to its exfoliation (loss) time, I agree that it would be rather silly to place a filling into a tooth that is waving in the breeze. If a tooth is painful and so badly rotted that it would be impossible to restore properly, extraction, rather than filling, might have to be considered. If a decayed tooth is not painful and not infected, it can be left in place (closely observed by the dentist) without filling until it loosens and is lost naturally.

The main reason to preserve baby teeth as long as practical (other than for chewing, of course) is to maintain space for the permanent teeth that replace the baby teeth. Primary teeth act as natural space maintainers, keeping jaw space available for the new teeth. They serve as guides, helping to direct permanent teeth into their correct positions. If a baby tooth must be lost early, your dentist may suggest that a spacer be made to hold that gap open, allowing the permanent tooth to erupt properly. So if a tooth can be restored, even though it's "only" a baby tooth, have it done.

Dental Exams

When should dental exams start? Anytime you, as a parent, are scheduled for an exam, bring the youngster with you. Two or three years old is not too young for the child to familiarize himself/herself with the dental office, if only for a ride in the chair and to get acquainted with the dentist and the equipment. I've been squirted in the face many times by the kids. They love the water/air syringe and their aim is quite good. Somewhere around four years old is a good time to start having regular dental examinations. It depends on the maturity of the child and whether the dentist will actually be able to take x-rays and perform a thorough examination.

I'll discuss dental exams in more detail when I talk about adults on page 22.

Fluoride

Putting political or religious issues aside (both outside my field), I'm a firm supporter of using fluoride in controlling tooth decay. Whether it is given in combination with vitamins or through water fluoridation, it is an indispensable adjunct to proper care of the teeth. The fluoride actually binds to and becomes part of the tooth structure itself.

It makes teeth harder and more impervious to decay.

Treatment can be started, with the approval of your dentist and/or pediatrician, at infancy, in the form of fluoride-containing liquid vitamins and can be completed at about age thirteen, when all the permanent teeth have finished erupting.

One-half part per million for infants and one part per million for children and young teenagers is the customary dosage. Many locations throughout the United States have sufficient fluoride within the water supply, and supplemental treatment may not be necessary. Check with your dentist. S/he should know.

All four of my children, three grown and one, age fourteen, were on fluoride supplements from infancy until they were about twelve years old. I don't believe that collectively there were four cavities amongst them (and, believe me, it wasn't due to good brushing habits).

An economic point of information: try to convince your dentist or pediatrician to prescribe the generic (non-brand name) form of the medication. It is far less expensive than its commercial relative.

Five to Thirteen Years

A mixed dentition is one in which there is a combination of baby and adult teeth present in the mouth. It's a rather awkward appearing stage that all children experience. Baby teeth are being lost and adult teeth are replacing them. The remaining baby teeth, until they come out, will appear dwarfed by the size of the permanent front teeth. I'm certain you have some memories of that gawky stage of life.

Eruption Dates of Permanent Teeth

As with baby teeth, eruption dates are only approximate. The sequence of eruption here is more important than it is for baby teeth. I'll go into the sequence of the erupting permanent teeth, as well as the average age of the youngsters, so that you'll have an idea when to expect the baby teeth to start loosening. There's a picture on the next page.

Improper eruption order of the adult dentition could cause crowding and might require future orthodontic treatment. If caught early enough, the problem might be made easier for the orthodontist. Your dentist should alert you. Don't be afraid to ask.

The first permanent teeth to erupt (and they are rather sneaky about it) are the six-year (first) molars. They come in at about six or seven years of age. Wouldn't you think that the first adult teeth to come in would be the front teeth, first loosening, then pushing the baby front teeth out? Not so. These tricksters erupt in the back part of the mouth, behind the baby second molars. No baby teeth are displaced at this time.

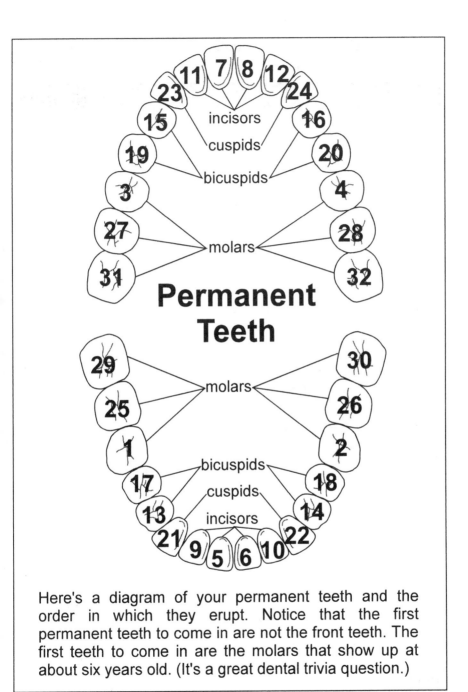

incisors

cuspids

bicuspids

molars

Permanent Teeth

molars

bicuspids

cuspids

incisors

Here's a diagram of your permanent teeth and the order in which they erupt. Notice that the first permanent teeth to come in are not the front teeth. The first teeth to come in are the molars that show up at about six years old. (It's a great dental trivia question.)

These new molars are usually the first of the adult dentition to decay, not necessarily because they are first in, but because eruption occurs with so little fuss that parents many times think these permanent molars are still baby teeth. Nothing was lost; nothing has happened. So why be concerned if a dark spot appears on the chewing surface? It's only a baby tooth, correct? Wrong. This is one of many reasons for having routine exams, starting at a very young age.

The six-year molars are followed by the front teeth (lower ones first, usually), pushing their baby equivalents out as they erupt. It's money time for the kids if the tooth fairy is still solvent. This takes place between six and eight years old. The side front teeth are next, coming in somewhere around seven, eight and nine years of age.

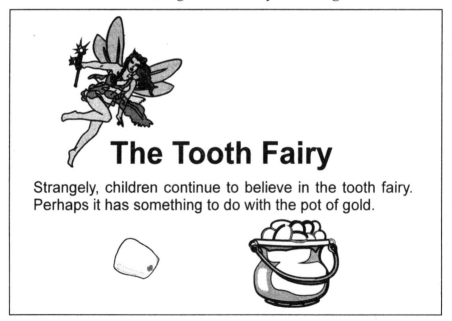

The Tooth Fairy

Strangely, children continue to believe in the tooth fairy. Perhaps it has something to do with the pot of gold.

The bicuspids come in anywhere between ten and twelve years old. Cuspids, canines, eyeteeth (all synonyms) show at about ten to thirteen years. Twelve-year (second) molars pop into position between eleven and thirteen years. If you are wondering what all of these teeth look like, see the picture below.

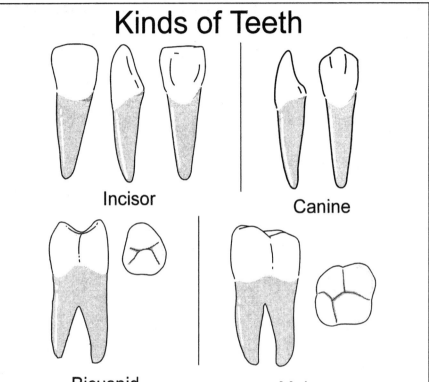

Kinds of Teeth

Incisor

Canine

Bicuspid

Molar

You have four kinds of teeth in your mouth (as long as you take care of them, that is): incisors, canines (or cuspids), bicuspids and molars. Did you know that cuspid means pointed? If you check your cuspid teeth, you'll notice that they have one point. Bicuspid teeth have two points. (Bi means two.) Your molars have four.

In the picture the white part of the tooth is covered with hard enamel. The gray part is covered with the softer cementum. Healthy gums cover up the tooth all the way to the enamel.

Spacing

Just as with primary teeth, there are multiple forces at work in the child's mouth when permanent teeth come in. Don't be too concerned if, initially, the front teeth aren't straight. If there is a space problem, there's not much that can be accomplished until most of the adult teeth have erupted. Your dentist will keep you informed.

Brushing

If you taught well when the baby teeth came in, proper brushing, by now, should be an everyday habit. Let's be realistic though. Brushing, to kids and young teens, no matter what anyone says, is a real nuisance. Whether it be one, two or three minutes, brushing takes away from their pleasure time. It won't hurt to nag and double-check once in a while. "Honey, don't forget to brush your teeth." "I won't, Ma, don't worry." You can always check the brush to see if it's moist. I don't think that the youngster is devious enough (yet) to consider wetting the toothbrush and putting it away without using it. Brushing after breakfast and after dinner should be mandatory. When children are at school, good luck; they're on their own.

Do you know when kids (children and teenagers alike) really learn the benefits of good home care? It'll hit like lightening out of the blue when they hear four words, loud and clear, from the dentist, "You have a cavity."

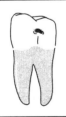

Cavity

Unfortunately, a cavity may be the only thing that convinces your children that brushing and flossing are worth the effort.

Chipped and Fractured Teeth

Accidents do happen. Chipping and fracturing of teeth can occur anytime during life, but it's more apt to happen between five years old and the early teens. Skateboard accidents, roller blades, bicycles, fights, you name it. Treatment depends on the severity and type of injury. More information on chipped and fractured teeth is covered in this book starting on page 40.

Mouth guards are like seatbelts for the teeth. They won't prevent accidents but, if kids wore them, the number of fractured teeth would certainly be minimized. The only question is, how on earth do you get invincible youngsters to wear the appliance?

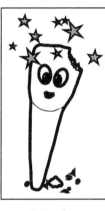

Chipped Teeth

Accidents do happen but there are ways to reduce the risk. Mouthguards for high risk activities such as skateboarding and contact sports are a common sense idea. Now try and convince your kids.

My fourteen year old is an avid skate boarder. He won't even wear a helmet or wrist guards, let alone an ugly mouth guard. It's just not cool. "Dad, I'm not going to fall and break anything. Why do you worry so much?" So far, thank goodness, he's kept his word. I'm a pushover. I strongly suggest that you be much stricter than I am.

Be firm about it. Don't allow participation without the proper protective gear. The kids will ultimately come around to your way of thinking. The earlier you start nagging, the better the likelihood that safety equipment will be used. Fractured teeth aren't cool either.

Teenagers

Eruption Dates of Permanent Teeth (Continued)

By adolescence we have most of our permanent teeth. Wisdom teeth (third molars), if they erupt at all, will do so somewhere between seventeen and twenty-one years of age. Interesting thing about wisdom teeth: through the process of evolution, mouths are getting smaller (although with some people, that's open to debate). Raw meat doesn't have to be ripped from bones as our pre-historic ancestors had to do. Our diet today consists of refined foods, much softer in their consistency. Therefore, Mother Nature has concluded that there's less need for these extra teeth. Fewer wisdom teeth buds are forming. Those that do form, in many instances, don't have room to erupt properly and remain as potential problems, impacted beneath the gums and bone (the oral surgeon's delight). There is more on problems with wisdom teeth on page 36.

That's it for eruption of permanent teeth. Twenty-eight in all (thirty-two, counting wisdom teeth), beginning to come in at about six years and being fully in position at thirteen years old (seventeen to twenty-one with wisdom teeth). See the picture of the teeth on the next page.

Oral Hygiene

Teenagers are far too busy to be bothered with dental appointments, let alone with brushing their teeth. Social and athletic activities generally predominate their lives and anything else is an imposition on their time. I would say that studying (usually forced) is a distant second. Who knows where tooth brushing enters into the priority picture.

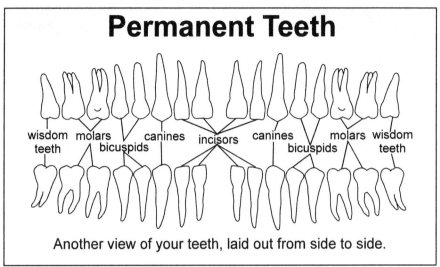

Permanent Teeth

wisdom teeth   molars   bicuspids   canines   incisors   canines   bicuspids   molars   wisdom teeth

Another view of your teeth, laid out from side to side.

Here's an important fact. *The decay rate of teeth is at its peak during the teen years.* This is not because teeth are physiologically more vulnerable during these formative years, but primarily because brushing habits and diet are far from ideal. It's a real problem. Even when teens do brush, it's a quick once over, rinse and goodbye. The front teeth are given far more attention than the back teeth because they are more visible, and teenagers are very appearance conscious. A nice white smile, therefore, doesn't really mean a cavity-free mouth.

If you have any ideas how to motivate teenagers to brush properly, please tell me. Logical explanations, fright, threat, grounding, bribes, all have some impact, but teens still have to be reminded continually (ah, the joys of parenthood). Older teens seem to be more conscientious. I suppose that's because they're approaching (as we adults all know) the wiser stage of life, adulthood.

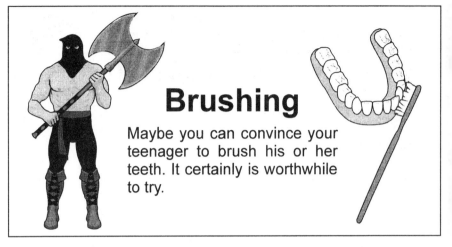

Brushing

Maybe you can convince your teenager to brush his or her teeth. It certainly is worthwhile to try.

Lack of brushing also creates an environment for gum irritation that can be the precursor to early stage periodontal disease. This is discussed at length, starting on page 69.

Adults

Dental Exams

Timely dental exams, x-rays and professional cleanings are essential for all age groups. I thought I would discuss them here because there is one aspect of dentistry created by the lack of thorough examination that occurs in adults only. Neither infants, nor children, nor teens suffer this particular problem. It's paying those high dental bills for everybody else.

Dentistry is expensive enough. Letting things go makes it even costlier. With exams every six to eight months, small cavities can be caught and cared for early, thus reducing the possibility of expensive, extensive treatment (and discomfort). The same non-disputable logic holds true for gum problems.

At the Dentists

We dentists are just nice, friendly folks who want to help you take care of your teeth. Come on in every six to eight months and we'll clean your teeth, check for cavities and make sure that everything else in your mouth is doing okay.

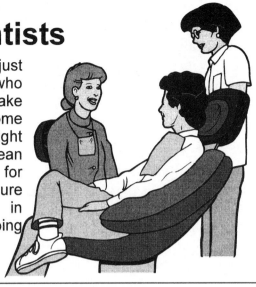

Dentists not only examine teeth, but they also check the status of the mouth in general: gums, cheeks, tongue, lips and throat. Clinical observation of oral conditions may facilitate early diagnosis of certain general health problems. Lip and mouth cancers also can be spotted in their earliest stages when the chance for a cure is very high.

Bridgework — Why and When

Bridges are nothing more than replacements for missing teeth. There are basically two types of bridges, fixed and removable. Removable bridges are usually referred to as partial dentures.

Bridges are placed when there are teeth missing. Caps are made for the teeth on either side of the space created by the lost tooth. A false tooth is welded between these caps and the entire appliance is cemented as one solid unit.

Bridges serve a number of purposes. Primarily, they replace function that is lost when teeth have been extracted. Bridges also serve to help maintain the integrity of the dental arch by preventing "caving in" of the remaining teeth into the space(s) created by extraction. In addition to the above, bridges, in those instances where teeth are lost close to the front of the mouth, can restore appearance, eliminating any gaps that might otherwise show.

Generally speaking, fixed bridges are more desirable than removable appliances simply because they become part of you and remain in position. They are cemented into place. The possibility of cement bonds breaking and bridgework falling out is minimal. There is little likelihood of damage to fixed bridges.

Some special care must be given to bridges. Cleanliness is important, but it's simple.

Have your dentist give you a "bridge cleaner," an appliance which you can use to clean the area under the false tooth that was welded between the caps. Other than that, only normal hygiene is necessary.

Removable partials are, by definition, teeth replacements that can be (and should be) removed daily for cleaning. One very big disadvantage to removable partials is that they are food traps. They *must* be removed to clean them properly. If cleaning (out of the mouth) is not routinely done, not only will the foulest of odors emanate from your mouth, but also cavities will most certainly form.

Removable partials serve the same purpose as their fixed counterparts. Most people consider them a nuisance or a necessary evil.

Breakage is more of a problem with this type of replacement as they are made of a combination of a rather brittle metal and acrylic. Metal breakage can be a difficult laboratory repair, while acrylic or tooth breakage can, in some cases, be quite easy to repair. (See the chapter on Dentures, starting on page 95.)

Fixed bridgework, tooth for tooth, is much more expensive than removable. It is, in most cases, also far superior to partial dentures.

A practical point for your consideration:

Ideally, when teeth are extracted, they *should* be replaced. If teeth are lost in early adulthood, undesirable movement and shifting of some of the remaining teeth can occur. If teeth have been missing for a long period of time, or if some extractions are necessary later in life, replacement, although desirable, may not be a necessity. Teeth adjacent to long-standing spaces usually have already experienced all the movement that will occur. If chewing is not a problem and appearance is not a concern, practically speaking, replacements may not be essential.

I'm sure I would get some arguments from practicing dentists on my realistic approach to the matter. Since I'm retired, however, I really have no axe to grind. I'm not losing business by trying to save someone a few dollars.

Seniors

Think about this simple fact. There are very few parts of the human body that maintain their integrity (don't naturally decay) as we age. Teeth are an excellent example. Enamel is the hardest tissue in the human body. Why then does a good percentage of the senior population wear full or partial dental plates?

Ideally, with proper dental care throughout life, senior dental problems should be no greater and, in many instances, will be less than in other age groups. The older generation's teeth are harder and their eating habits are much better. The operative word here is "ideally."

Gum Shrinkage

Since the gums have a tendency to recede somewhat with aging (as do hairlines), seniors must be a bit more conscientious when brushing (teeth not hair). As gum shrinkage occurs, more tooth root is exposed in the mouth. Roots are not covered with hard enamel that encompasses the crowns of teeth. They are covered by a much softer material called cementum that, by virtue of its texture, is more prone to cavities if not properly cleaned.

There is a myth that has been floating around for many years that no matter what is done to maintain your teeth, there comes a time when loss will occur regardless of the care that has been taken. So why bother to spend money on exams and cleanings and fillings, when the teeth will be goners anyway?

There may have been some basis for this belief in years past. The present senior population, when younger, didn't have the luxury of the advanced preventative and corrective techniques that are available today. The importance of proper dental hygiene and the subsequent consequences of insufficient home and professional care were not adequately emphasized in generations past.

This "semi-fairytale" has caused the unnecessary loss of many teeth in those people who would latch onto any excuse, rational or not, to stay away from dentists. The simple fact is that losing teeth most certainly is *not* part of the natural aging process.

The majority of teeth that have to be extracted on adults and seniors (contrary to popular belief) are lost because of gum and bone disease, not because of decay. In some instances, the patient is not to blame. Many dentists, unfortunately, have a tendency to overlook gum disease. It's easy to do. Gum and bone disease develop slowly and insidiously, many times with few, if any, symptoms. If cleanings are not routinely and properly done over the years and if the spaces between the teeth and gums are not regularly observed and measured professionally, gum disease can occur and will lead to tooth loss. Caught early, gum disease can be treated with relative ease. Caught late, it's usually *too* late. Short of having to undergo gum and bone surgery, some teeth will probably be lost.

Bad Breath and Getting Older

Bad breath is associated with advancing years. It can occur at any age with lack of proper oral hygiene, but seniors are more susceptible to the problem because their salivary glands don't function quite the way they used to (what does?). If the mouth is dry and saliva doesn't wash away normal mouth bacteria, unbelievable odors can seep out. Inexpensive, over-the-counter saliva substitutes can be purchased to minimize this potential problem.

Dentures can also cause bad breath. Since they are made of a porous material, bacteria can invade and flourish. Proper cleaning can minimize the problem.

Chapter 3: Teeth

Baby Bottle Decay

Baby gets a good diet and is obviously not eating candies or junk food like you and I do, so how can cavities form so rapidly in an infant's teeth?

Many parents allow their child to fall asleep sucking on a bottle of milk or juice. This may act as a pacifier and help put baby to sleep, but it's the worst thing in the world for their little teeth. The sugar in the liquid stays in the mouth all night long because swallowing occurs much less frequently while asleep. This allows the mouth to dry out, and the bacteria that are nourished by the sugar can rapidly decay the teeth. This occurs much more frequently than you might imagine.

Baby Bottles at Bedtime

A sleeping baby is a wonderful thing, but giving a baby a bottle of milk or juice at bedtime is just asking for trouble with the baby's teeth. The sugar in either milk or juice is a leading cause of tooth decay in babies. A bottle of water or a pacifier is a better way to go.

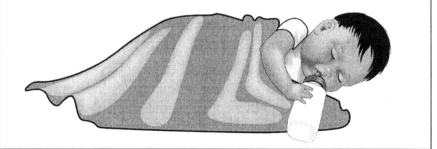

Nothing more need be said. Milk and juices are excellent for baby, but at the proper times. Bedtime is not one of those times unless the bottle is removed after the baby is asleep.

You can't treat the decay after it has developed. You must see the dentist for that. You can, however, definitely minimize the probability of its occurrence.

When it's baby's bedtime and you want to use something to calm baby down, try to use a plain pacifier. If the baby is well fed prior to bedtime, it's the sucking reflex that soothes and pacifies the infant. A bottle with water in it will also serve the same purpose. By the way, the same thing holds true during the waking hours. If the baby must have a bottle in his possession all day long, let it be water!

Pacifiers are one of those double-edged swords. On one hand they can mellow out the baby, but on the other hand they can cause severe bite or speech problems that may well require tooth straightening in the future. If you insist on your baby's using the pacifier beyond the age of two or three, save lots of money for the orthodontist or speech therapist. Keep an extra pacifier for yourself later on, when the bills start coming in.

Sensitive Teeth

Sensitivity in the teeth can be caused by a number of things. It does not always mean that you have cavities, although that is a possibility.

There are four major types of sensitivity associated with teeth. They are temperature sensitivity, sweet sensitivity, pressure sensitivity and a combination of the above. In many cases, people are sensitive to more than one thing. The type of sensitivity gives the dentist some clues about what is wrong with the tooth.

Sensitivity to cold indicates a number of conditions, ranging from new fillings to cavities and many points in between.

If the teeth become sensitive right after they are filled, this can be considered normal. The sensitivity should subside within a few days, although it could last up to a couple of weeks. It should let up without any treatment being necessary. This type of sensitivity is due to the heat created by the rotating drill's irritation of the nerve. It takes the nerve a while to calm down.

Another cold sensitivity is caused by the gums shrinking back, which leaves the root portion of the tooth exposed. This can be extremely sensitive because the roots of the teeth have very little protection between them and the nerves enclosed within. This is readily handled by using desensitizing toothpaste or, if that doesn't work, by a simple procedure done by your dentist.

Go out and buy some "desensitizing" toothpaste and use it routinely. After you finish brushing, take a dab of the paste, put it on your fingertip and rub it onto the areas of the teeth, most often near the gum line, that are sensitive. Let your saliva wash that toothpaste away.

This treatment will not give instant relief. It must be done over a period of about two weeks. Results vary for different people. As best, expect about a sixty to seventy percent reduction of sensitivity. If it works for you and you adore the taste, you can use it routinely as your regular toothpaste.

If this is not successful, there is a simple procedure that your dentist can perform. He will place a desensitizing solution onto the offending teeth and, with two or three quick treatments, can effectively put an end to, or at least minimize, your having to drink warm beer.

Discomfort from heat usually indicates a more serious problem. It could be symptomatic of an abscessing tooth (a tooth that has an infection in the bone or tissue surrounding the root).

Abscessed teeth can be excruciatingly painful to pressure. Here, either extraction or root canal therapy must be done. *There are no other alternatives when abscessed teeth are present.*

Sensitivity to sweets is a good indication that there is a cavity forming. If *any* food (regardless of taste type) gets into the cavity, you bet you'll feel it. Cavities and decaying teeth usually respond unfavorably to both cold and sweet. The sensitivity will not subside without dental treatment.

Pressure sensitive teeth can be caused by an incorrect bite when a new filling has not been properly contoured. This situation can be corrected by having your dentist trim some filling material away, allowing teeth to contact each other properly. Another cause of pressure sensitive teeth is continual clenching of the jaws. See night grinding on page 121 for some treatment options.

Cracked teeth may demonstrate any or all of these symptoms. See the next section. Periodontally involved teeth may also demonstrate a mixed bag of symptoms. See the discussion of gum problems in Chapter 4.

Any sensitivity that does not subside on its own, or with self-treatment, within one or two weeks (usually time enough for new filling sensitivity to quiet down) should get you on your way to the dentist. Letting it go longer will only create a greater problem for both you and the dentist. Don't be an ostrich. Hiding your head exposes other vulnerable parts.

Cracked Teeth

Chipped teeth are visually obvious. When they are located, they can usually (depending on the severity of the chip) be treated successfully by your dentist without too much difficulty. (See page 40.)

Hairline cracks within the tooth structure itself may *not* be visible and, in many cases, cannot be seen in x-rays or during a routine oral exam. They present, in many instances, a complex diagnostic problem for the dentist as well as a source of nondescript sensitivity for the patient.

A cracked tooth can initially manifest itself as a slightly cold sensitive tooth. Over a period of time (anywhere from weeks to months to years) symptoms can become more severe. Ultimately the tooth may become extremely sensitive, not only to cold, but to pressure as well. This change, if it occurs, and the increasing severity of discomfort are indications that the crack is gradually and progressively worsening.

Sometimes, even at the height of the discomfort, no visible cause for the pain can be found until it's too late (seeing mobility when the tooth has totally split into two parts). Unfortunately, at that point the tooth quite probably will have to be extracted.

If the crack is found early on, it is possible to correct the problem. A cap and perhaps a root canal treatment *may* resolve the situation. The only way to find out, if in fact your symptoms are so severe, is to have the dentist start these procedures. It could be costly, and may be to no avail.

Don't forget that economic practicality may have to dictate what treatment you undergo. It's unfortunate, but it's a fact of life.

Toothache

There aren't many pains that are worse than a toothache. Some first aid ideas that will help ease the pain until you get to a dentist (and you *are* going to a dentist) include cool water directly on the tooth, teething medicine and oil of cloves. Taking aspirin can help, too. And remember, even if the pain goes away, you still need to see a dentist right away!

Toothache

When we talk about a toothache, we are talking about a throbbing pain with possible jaw swelling, not just simple sensitivity to cold or sweet. The dental first aid covered here is only temporary, until you can see the dentist.

There are very few words or thoughts that can conjure up an adequate description of an honest-to-goodness, old-fashioned, excruciating, intolerable, pounding, throbbing, nerve-wracking toothache. The amplification of the sound of fingernails screeching on a blackboard might come close. Someone clubbing your head repeatedly with a sledgehammer, after you've had a night on the town, might approximate the sensation.

When things get this far out of hand, the tooth or teeth involved are going to require some type of extensive, expensive treatment, ranging from a nerve treatment or root canal, along with the fabrication of a cap, to an extraction. You are very likely dealing with a deeply decayed, severely infected tooth.

Prescription pain pills, if available, will definitely help. If a prescription is not feasible, aspirin is terrific for toothaches. If there are no allergies, swallow the aspirin with some water. Take two, every four to six hours. Do not think that placing the aspirin near the tooth and letting it dissolve in the area will help. It won't, I give you my solemn word on that one. All you will succeed in doing is burning the gums.

If there is an infection involved, cool to cold water directly over the tooth can be very effective. It is not the best thing for the infection; but we're talking pain relief *right now*, and the cold water can do the trick. As a matter of fact, this might be just as beneficial as pain pills, if not better. The relief can be immediate but will last only as long as you keep cold water in your mouth. Mind you, this is only for that pulsating, throbbing, miserable toothache that is so bad it makes you want to die and, what's even worse, you know that you aren't going to.

The use of cold water is not for the sensitivity that you might experience due to sweets and/or cold caused by a cavity or by receding gums. Quite the contrary, cold water on that type of sensitivity can shoot you right through the roof as though someone stuck a rocket under your rear end.

Another effective remedy for toothache is oil of cloves. This medication has a sedative action on the nerves of the teeth and can be very effective in reducing the pain to a dull roar. All you need do is to place a few drops onto the problem tooth. This should handle the pain until you see the dentist. No prescription is necessary. This stuff, by the way, has the smell that most people associate with a dental office. It is used when the dentist mixes temporary, sedative-type fillings. Now there's a bit of fantastic, yet totally useless, dental knowledge.

Any teething medicine can help. They all have benzo-caine, which is a topical anesthetic, as their main active in-gredient. The deeper the cavity in the tooth, the better this type of treatment works. Just smear some over the entire area, tooth and gums. Again, no prescription is required.

By the way, the fact that the pain might subside with self-treatment doesn't by any stretch of the imagination mean that the problem is solved. Infected teeth can rot down to the gum line with minimal pain. At its absolute worst, an untreated abscessed tooth can be life threatening. Don't for-get: it's an infection and like any other infection, it can spread. Go see a dentist and have it taken care of!

Wisdom Tooth (Third Molar) Pain

Wisdom teeth don't always erupt totally when starting to move around. The picture on the next page shows how this can happen. Many times they won't erupt at all or will only partially come in. If they decide not to erupt, they might just move around under the gums and bone for short periods of time, causing temporary, mild discomfort. Then the teeth may stop moving and can remain nice and quiet for years.

This situation is obviously caused by a wisdom tooth that is starting to move around under the bone and gums. It can also be caused by an already partially erupted wisdom tooth that is moving further into the mouth.

A good percentage of wisdom-tooth pain is caused by the tooth's pushing the gums upward, causing irritation and swelling. When the gums become swollen, the teeth oppos-ing that area, in the opposite arch, will further irritate those already puffy gums by biting on them, causing them to swell even more. It becomes a nasty, vicious circle.

Impacted Wisdom Teeth

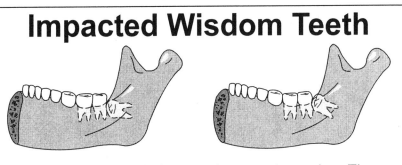

Sometimes those wisdom teeth are not so wise. These pictures show what happens when wisdom teeth do not have enough room in the jaw to come in properly. The tooth on the left is still inside the jaw bone. The one on the right can be felt in the gum or may be just breaking through the gum. Neither of the teeth is doing anything good for the molars in front of it or for your general comfort.

A wisdom tooth that has partially poked its way into the mouth can cause more problems than one that is still totally under the gums. Food particles can work their way down between the tooth and the gum. These particles become very difficult to remove, causing quite an irritation/infection. Vigorous rinsing is very helpful in flushing out the debris that gets caught. Sorry about the word "flushing," but it's properly descriptive. The forceful rinsing serves the same purpose as pushing the little handle on the toilet. It cleans out the contents.

To rinse, make a mixture with equal amounts of warm water and hydrogen peroxide solution. Rinse the area energetically. This will serve two purposes. First, it will help wash out any junk that may have lodged under the gums around the wisdom tooth and, second, it will help to pull out the inflammation and reduce the swelling in the gums. Do this for two or three days, as many times each day as is practical. Four, six, ten times each day, I don't care. And remember, it's best not to swallow this mixture.

Any teething medicine that contains benzocaine will be helpful. Place a dab over the sore gums. This should numb the area sufficiently to reduce the discomfort. Obviously, if things don't quiet down within a few days, you'll get to the dentist.

If possible, keep to a soft diet and try to keep from chomping down on the affected area. That's it. Pain pills of course, if necessary, can also be used.

If you have continual problems with irritated gums in the wisdom tooth area and if the dentist feels that the tooth will be coming into a comparatively normal position, he can perform a relatively routine procedure by removing that extra gum tissue overlying the tooth. It'll be quick, inexpensive and relatively painless. With this accomplished, the wisdom tooth can fully erupt into its position quite rapidly. Wisdom teeth that have fully erupted can be solid, functional teeth for life.

Extracting Wisdom Teeth

There are varying opinions as to whether or not wisdom teeth should be routinely extracted. Oral surgeons will almost always suggest extraction. As a matter of fact, many surgeons will suggest removal of all the wisdom teeth. Their rationale is simple and does have some validity. Those teeth, when not properly erupted, are very definitely *potential* sources of infection.

This line of reasoning is difficult to dispute. Be mindful, though, that oral surgeons do make their living primarily by extracting teeth. Their opinion, therefore, might be slightly biased. It's not wrong, but it might be somewhat aggressive.

Orthodontists may want you to consider having your third molars extracted if they feel that they are applying undue pressure to the teeth in front of them.

This pressure might have a tendency to shift those teeth that your orthodontist so tediously, meticulously and expensively straightened over the years. This potential problem does not happen often and can usually be spotted early on in x-rays.

Many good-old-fashioned general dentists, of which I am one (very old), will tell you: if they don't bother you, you don't bother them. If the wisdom teeth don't annoy you and if the discomfort is minimal and infrequent, please insert one of the following sayings:

1. Don't create problems that don't exist.

2. Let a sleeping dog lie.

3. Don't stir up a hornet's nest.

4. Why change a good thing.

5. If it ain't broke, don't fix it

All of the above are quite valid.

If the third molars should happen to bother you more than two or three times a year, they could be causing some damage to the teeth directly in front of them. Serious consideration should then be given to the unpleasant possibility of extraction. You should at least visit the dentist to determine if he feels that extractions are necessary. As I said before, this damage, if any, can be determined by having x-rays taken of the areas that are bothering you.

Does anyone know, or does anyone care to know, why they are called wisdom teeth? If you are really a trivia buff, it's because they erupt later in life, usually in adulthood, when, as we all know, we are much wiser.

Chipped Baby Tooth

(Usually a front tooth.) First of all, don't panic. Then control any bleeding from the lip area. (See page 73 for "Bleeding in and around the Mouth and Lips.") If there is no pain involved and there are no sharp edges, things can wait until you make an appointment to see your dentist. He will probably just smooth over any roughness with a small sandpaper disk and that's that. No pain, no strain and no shot. You might even be able to do it yourself with an emery board. Don't forget, the baby front teeth are usually lost between ages five and seven years, so a small chip is only temporary until a permanent tooth replaces the broken baby tooth. Really, no big deal.

If there's a large break and you can see a pink spot in the center of the tooth, that's an indication that the fracture has gone into the nerve. The pink spot is the blood supply to the tooth. This can be very painful as the nerve and blood vessels are both located in the same channel within the tooth. Use baby aspirin or baby Tylenol and get to the dentist fast.

Important note: Do not place aspirin on the tooth or on the gums near the tooth. Have the child swallow the pill with warm water, because cold water might cause quite a bit of sensitivity. Naturally, use the chewable or liquid baby medication if pill swallowing can't be tolerated.

Putting aspirin over the tooth or gums will do nothing more than hurt the tooth and quite probably burn the gums. Don't forget, aspirin is an acid. See the dentist as soon as possible.

Broken Teeth

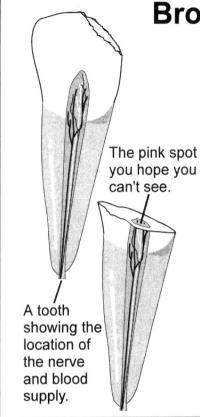

The pink spot you hope you can't see.

A tooth showing the location of the nerve and blood supply.

First of all, stay calm. Control any bleeding from the lip area. Then check the tooth.

The top picture shows a broken tooth where the nerve is still all right. If there is no pain and you can't feel any sharp edges, you can wait to make an appointment to see your dentist.

If the break gets down to the nerve, you will see a pink spot in the center of the tooth. The bottom picture shows the nerve area on the top of the tooth. This is an emergency. You need to get to a dentist fast.

If the break is large and you see that pink spot, there is definitely a nerve exposure to the baby tooth. A decision then has to be made by both you and the dentist. Do you have the tooth extracted? Does the dentist do a nerve treatment? How wealthy are you? Treatment also depends on the age of the child. If the youngster is near the age when this tooth is slated to fall out, there is no reason whatsoever to save the tooth. You should consider having it pulled. If the child is younger, then some consideration might be given to having the nerve treatment done, not because of a potential future space problem, but primarily because of appearance.

Rarely is there a problem with the space closing up when a front baby tooth is lost early. If the front permanent tooth was going to erupt into its proper position, it will do so, even with the baby tooth being lost prematurely. If you opt to have the tooth extracted, a skilled dentist should be able to remove the tooth without undue discomfort. There will be an injection involved. If the dentist has the capability, it would be a good idea for him or her to pre-medicate the youngster before giving the shot. This will serve to calm the dentist as well as the patient. A relaxed patient translates to a relaxed dentist and vice versa. If the dentist suggests a nerve removal, let him do it. It could be less traumatic to the child than an extraction and the tooth can be retained. It may darken a bit but, again, this tooth is ultimately going to be replaced by the permanent tooth.

Some type of basic restoration should be placed on the involved tooth. Restoring the full contour of the tooth is really not necessary.

Chipped Permanent Tooth

(Usually a front tooth.) Control any bleeding around the mouth. (See page 73 for "Bleeding in and around the Mouth and Lips.")

Unfortunately, I can't give you much first aid help here. If the chip is small and there is little or no sensitivity, you might be able to smooth any rough edges with an emery board, but that's about it. You can use some beeswax to cover the area if you are experiencing some sensitivity. Get to the dentist for treatment.

Some type of restoration will have to be done profession-ally. Naturally, on a front tooth, appearance is all important. You'll want to get in to the dental office as soon as possible to prevent any further damage to the tooth and to cover that unsightly chip.

With only a small fracture, there's a good possibility that an expensive laboratory-processed cap will not be necessary. There are tooth-colored filling materials available that are excellent in appearance and durability. The stability of the filling is in direct relation to the size of the fracture. The fillings are far less expensive than the caps.

With a large chip, a filling may still be able to be done, but it will not be quite as strong as the smaller restoration. Even large fillings, however, with today's bonding techniques and materials, are rather strong.

If there is nerve involvement along with the chip, believe me, you'll be in the dentist's office in a flash. (See the picture on page 41 for an explanation of how to check for nerve damage.) Very probably a root canal and a cap will both be necessary. Very expensive, sorry.

Baby Tooth Knocked Out, Lips Lacerated

Please stay calm. Your attitude will definitely be conveyed to the youngster. First control the bleeding. (See page 73 for "Bleeding in and around the Mouth and Lips.")

As for the tooth or teeth involved, if the child is three, four and even an early five year old, the teeth are almost certainly baby teeth. If they are knocked out completely, don't even worry about looking for them. Forget them. Remember, they will be replaced by the adult teeth. Do see the dentist. Let him, if possible, take an x-ray of the area, to make certain that if a tooth was lost, it came out in its entirety.

If a baby tooth has to be lost early, either knocked out or extracted, a front tooth is of the least importance. The front part of the mouth, usually the upper, is where most accidents occur. Baby falls smack on his face and an upper front tooth is loosened or knocked out.

If the teeth are just slightly loosened and not lost (this holds true for both baby and permanent teeth), they will, more often than not, tighten up on their own. The dentist may have to do a bit of repositioning along with some splinting and bonding, but with minimal care those loosened teeth should ultimately be fine.

A lost front baby tooth does not have to be replaced. I don't care what anyone says. It's only a temporary appearance problem and all kids go through that stage. It will probably bother the parents more than it will the child. Don't even think about a replacement. The child has already been through enough, don't you think?

There's one potential problem with a front baby tooth being knocked out. When the dentist takes an x-ray (and he should do so, if it's feasible), if the picture shows that part of the root of the tooth is still in its socket, this obviously means that the tooth was not totally knocked out. It has fractured off under the level of the gums. The dentist may then have to extract that remaining root tip. Unfortunately, your choices in this case are limited.

You might, however, consider this. If the root fragment is relatively solid, the dentist might suggest "watching and waiting." If the area is allowed to heal and the root remnant remains quiet, you may be able to wait until the permanent tooth that is slated to erupt into that position pushes that root fragment out. This can eliminate the trauma of the dentist's having to dig out that root part. If your dentist doesn't suggest this, don't hesitate to question him about the possibility. Your input is important.

The relative unimportance of the early loss of front baby teeth is not the case with premature loss of the back teeth. There can definitely be space closure. The teeth on either side of the lost tooth can tip and rotate into the void created. This tipping will partially close the space and may not allow the permanent tooth to erupt into its proper location. This is why, when there are cavities involved, the back baby teeth should be filled, rather than just pulled. If they must be pulled early, spacers can be easily and painlessly made to hold the space open until the permanent tooth comes in. The only pain involved will be to your bank account.

The necessity for a spacer is dependent on the child's age and how close to the surface the new tooth is. One simple x-ray can determine this. It would be foolish to make a spacer if the permanent tooth is due to erupt within a few months, so don't spend money if not necessary. That would be centsless.

Knocked-Out Permanent Tooth, With Lacerated Lips

It is usually a front tooth that is knocked out either by an accident such as falling from a skateboard or from a fight (which may or may not have been an accident).

The time factor here is *super* important. The sooner you get to the dentist, the better the chance of the dentist's being able to save the tooth and replant it into its socket.

The bleeding that usually goes hand in hand with the traumatic loss of a front tooth can readily be controlled by using a damp cold cloth, held with moderate pressure over lip lacerations. (See page 73 for "Bleeding in and around the Mouth and Lips.")

Knocked-Out Teeth

If a tooth is knocked all the way out, you must get to a dentist immediately! You have better than an eighty percent chance of saving the tooth if you get there within a half hour.

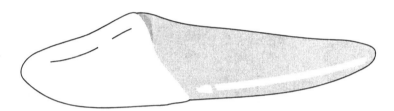

First of all, don't panic. Hold a cold cloth against the mouth to stop any bleeding. Find the tooth and rinse it in warm tap water. Don't scrub it. It will reattach better if you don't. Have the person hold it in his or her mouth under the tongue or wrap it in damp tissue. It's even better if you can put the tooth back in the socket but this can be hard (and painful) to do. Whatever you do, make sure the tooth doesn't get swallowed! Again, get to a dentist fast.

Finding a tooth lying on the ground is a great way to see what the root of a tooth really looks like. Unfortunately, you have other priorities.

You must find and rinse the tooth with warm tap water. Do *not* scrub, just rinse. It will attach better if the fibers are left on the root. Then, either wrap the tooth in gauze or tissue moistened with warm tap water or, even better, put the tooth back in the mouth and keep it under the tongue. It needs to be kept moist.

If the tooth can be repositioned into its socket, go ahead and do so; or at least try. Obviously, extreme care must be taken not to swallow the tooth. Don't waste too much time on this. *Get to a dentist as soon as possible.*

If you can get in to see the dentist within about a half an hour after the accident, your chances of having the tooth successfully replanted are between eighty and ninety percent. Not bad odds.

This could be a rather expensive treatment, requiring the removal of the nerve from within the tooth and filling the canal where the nerve was located with a sterile, rubber-like material. This is basically a procedure with which I'm sure you are familiar. At least you've heard about it. It's called root canal treatment. Wicked sounding, isn't it? If anything good can be said about root canals, this one will be done while the tooth is out of the mouth and will be, I guarantee, totally painless. However, the pain to your pocketbook will more than make up for the lack of physical pain.

The tooth, after the root canal is finished, can be repositioned into its socket. The dentist will then bond the injured tooth to the adjacent teeth for support, allowing the bone to heal and regenerate itself around the victim tooth. At a later date this bonding material can be removed.

Unfortunately, at some stage of the procedure, it will most likely be necessary to give an injection of local anesthetic to numb the area. Repositioning the tooth, in many instances, has to be done using a good deal of pressure and it's not the most pleasant sensation in the world.

The tooth may not last forever. Something happens and the root has a tendency to slowly shrink away. One case I recall that I did (and as far as I know is still intact), was completed about ten years ago. The follow-up x-rays showed some signs of root shrinkage but, to date, it's still a functioning tooth. I did a good job and so did the patient.

The parents got the boy into my office within fifteen minutes. I did the root canal treatment while holding the tooth in my hand. It took all of five to ten minutes, maximum. The tooth was then placed back into its socket and splinted to place. Yes, I do pat myself on the back once in a while, when I deserve it. I also yell at myself too, when I deserve that.

Loss of a Cap or Crown

If a cap should pop off, use a bit of denture adhesive paste. Have your dentist give you a small sample tube at the time he cements your caps. Squeeze some of the adhesive into the cap and then re-seat it over the remaining ugly stub of a tooth that you so desperately want to hide. It should be sticky enough to stay for a while. Re-apply adhesive as needed. Fill the hollow part of the cap with the adhesive. This material does not harden, so you won't damage the cap. Don't worry if you put too much in. The excess will just squish out in your mouth and can easily be cleaned away with your tongue. Swallowing it is no big deal either. I'm talking about swallowing the adhesive, *not the cap* — I'll address that problem shortly.

If denture adhesive isn't readily available, you can try to reseat the cap without the use of anything. Sometimes friction alone, between the tooth and cap, will be sufficient to retain the cap.

Make your necessary phone call and appointment. This is usually a routine, simple job for the dentist. Expense will be from zero to about $60, depending on the circumstances involved. I rarely charged for recementing any caps that I originally made. That was my guideline. If another dentist made the cap, I would impose a charge.

Losing a Cap

This is what you will (hopefully) find in your mouth when you lose a cap. Wash it off and put some denture adhesive in the hole.

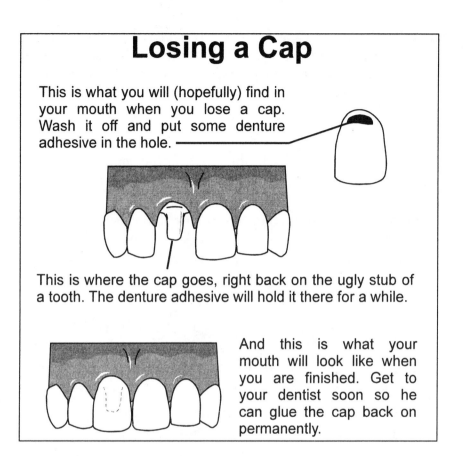

This is where the cap goes, right back on the ugly stub of a tooth. The denture adhesive will hold it there for a while.

And this is what your mouth will look like when you are finished. Get to your dentist soon so he can glue the cap back on permanently.

I use the term "cap" to indicate a laboratory-processed, tooth-shaped replacement that is cemented over the remaining part of your own tooth. Laboratory-processed caps, which cost a small fortune, do come off from time to time. Unfortunately, nothing is quite as durable as your own natural teeth. At any rate, if this cap that cost you a bundle, comes off, go buy some "stickum" and temporarily re-seat it. The stickum is any type of denture adhesive, paste preferred over the powder type.

Murphy's law prevails here. This will occur at the absolute worst possible time. It'll happen when you're on a first date, or at some type of social function, or just before a speech that you have to give at a dental convention. It would be bad enough if it happened to a back tooth, but Murphy insists that it be a front tooth and it will make you look exactly like Alfred E. Newman, of *Mad Magazine* fame.

Don't forget to go to the dentist for a permanent recementation. If it is a back tooth cap, don't leave it out of your mouth for more than a day or so. If you do, the involved tooth, as well as the teeth on either side of it and above it, can shift around in the mouth, making it very difficult, if not impossible, for the dentist to properly refit the cap. This holds true for the front teeth also, but people are more apt to get to the dental office right away if a front tooth is involved, simply because of the appearance.

When I was in practice, I had a couple of hard and fast rules that I always gave to my patients after I finished cementing a beautiful and, yes, expensive cap. No taffy, no Gummy Bears and don't chomp down into hard candies.

I was sitting at my desk one morning, before starting my workday, and a call came in from an obviously distressed and desperate patient. She was a school teacher whose cap had come out while she was getting ready for work. My receptionist told her to come right in and we would recement the cap for her.

You have to understand, this lady was a long time patient, an intelligent person, with a good sense of humor. She came in smiling broadly. I therefore knew immediately that it wasn't a front cap that had come off. The smile, however, was more of an embarrassed type of grin. "What happened?" I asked. Without so much as a word, she went inside her purse, still smiling, and dutifully took out the cap. It was firmly embedded in a delicious looking Mrs. See's caramel sucker. Then the patient laughed and in a quiet voice, almost apologetic in tone, she said something about having just lectured to her students about listening and following instructions.

I cleaned out the cap after extracting it from the sucker, recemented it, which was no big deal and gave her a few instructions again. No taffy, no Gummy Bears, etc. Get the picture? Besides, who on this earth eats caramel suckers for breakfast? Teachers?

Cap Swallowed (Gulp)

What if you are eating a super meal and your cap pops off and becomes part of that meal? Yes, I mean what if you swallow it?

There are two things you might do. One, if successful, can give immediate results. The other would be delayed. Can you guess?

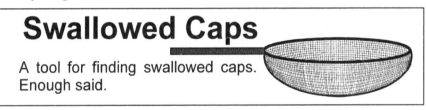

Swallowed Caps

A tool for finding swallowed caps. Enough said.

You could make yourself throw up. Preferably leave the dinner table first and hope that the cap will come up. I don't really recommend this type of treatment, but if you must do it, use the sink with the drain closed, rather than using the toilet. The cap is less apt to be lost. You will naturally have to fish around and try to locate it. I suggest using a strainer, if available, otherwise use your hand. This will definitely help you to throw up some more, in case the cap didn't come up the first time. Obviously this is not too pleasant a task, but if it's a front cap, because of the appearance, you just might consider it. At least that way, if it's retrieved, you can clean the cap and replace it in your mouth temporarily, as we discussed before.

The other method of retrieval will take longer, but it will be equally unpleasant. Check your stool. Not the sofa, not the chair, but your stool. If anything good can be said about this technique, it's reasonably under your control. This time please use the toilet rather than the sink.

Start with bowel movement number one. Sounds like a piano concerto, doesn't it? Again, use a strainer on your search. It'll make things a little easier on you. Continue checking for three to five days until it is retrieved. If it doesn't show up by then, it would be best to have your physician order an x-ray to determine the location of the cap.

Naturally, go to your dentist and have a temporary cap placed while your detective work is going on. When you finally retrieve your cap (and chances are pretty good that you will), you'll have to return to see the dentist again for a permanent recementation. I'm rather certain he'll have some distasteful jokes for you about your cap and its temporary home that won't be appreciated.

If you don't want to be the butt of his jokes, lie to him. Tell him it was stolen by a space alien and as they were taking off they dropped it or something equally as unbelievable. I really don't advocate lying to your health care professional but, in this case, I would probably do the same thing.

Don't forget, the cap will be thoroughly sterilized before replacement and will be as good as new. If you are contemplating not having it re-cemented because of the thought of where it was, try thinking about the $600 you'll have to shell out for a new cap. That should make some sense and, besides, what a terrific conversation piece.

Bridge that Fell Out

It's extremely rare that a bridge will fall out. If it does, it's just like two caps stuck together with another tooth in the middle. Use a little denture adhesive in each cap and get in to see your dentist for a permanent reattachment.

Particle of Food, Sliver from a Toothpick or Just a "Something" Wedged Between Your Teeth

First try vigorous rinsing. This probably won't work, but sometimes the pressure of squishing the water between the teeth will actually force the unwanted particle out.

If the rinsing doesn't help, dental floss is great for a problem like this. Snap the floss in between the problem teeth. Take it to the level of the gums or slightly under the gum level. Then slide the floss up and down along the sides of the involved teeth. You will be able to get under the object and loosen it. Then slide, don't snap, the floss out. After that, rinse thoroughly and forcefully to allow any remaining debris to be flushed away.

If neither rinsing nor flossing does the job, go to the pharmacy and buy some Stimudents. They come in a package that looks very much like a book of matches.

There are about thirty of them in a package. I love these things. They are glorified, modified toothpicks with a couple of important differences. First, they are made of a soft, balsa-type wood and, second, they are triangular shaped to fit properly between the teeth. Read the directions. Really, they don't require a college degree to use. Even I can do it.

Suck on the Stimudent for a few seconds to soften the wood. Place the pointed end between the involved teeth, flat side toward the gums. If the debris is lodged between lower

teeth, angle slightly downward. If the problem is on the upper, then you would angle slightly upward. Push forward
and you will almost certainly be at the proper level to force
out the foreign object.

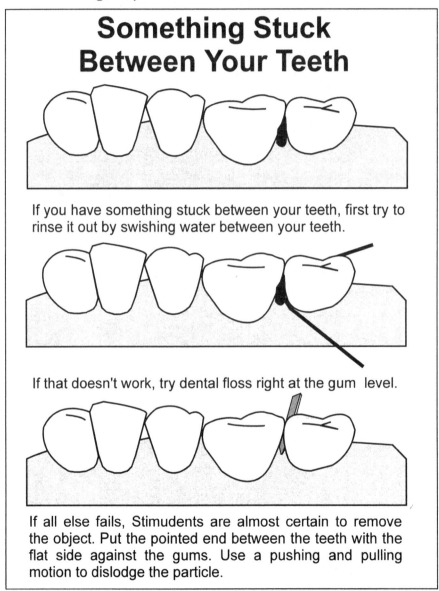

Something Stuck
Between Your Teeth

If you have something stuck between your teeth, first try to
rinse it out by swishing water between your teeth.

If that doesn't work, try dental floss right at the gum level.

If all else fails, Stimudents are almost certain to remove
the object. Put the pointed end between the teeth with the
flat side against the gums. Use a pushing and pulling
motion to dislodge the particle.

With a pulling and pushing motion, the pushing movement being the more pronounced, I'll bet you a dollar to a doughnut that you will succeed in removing the garbage. If I lose, use the Stimudent to remove any doughnut remaining between your teeth. I bet the doughnut; you bet the dollar.

The Stimudents are a great improvement over ordinary toothpicks. I use them myself after brushing if I'm too lazy to floss. They are terrific to help strengthen and firm the gums. Be consistent. Even if you don't have anything lodged between your teeth, you can do this at least once or twice daily. Place the Stimudent between the teeth and jiggle it back and forth a few times with slight pressure towards the gums. Start at the top back and go between all the teeth, top and bottom. It takes only a minute or so and it will really do you some good. In the long run it will most definitely help keep your dental bills down. Isn't that what we all want?

Lost Filling, Tooth Sensitive to Cold or Sweet

The first aid is very temporary, but very effective.

If you have any beeswax or candles around the house, soften the wax and place a bit into the hole that was created by the lost filling, which, for some reason, always feels as though you can drive a truck through it with room to spare.

A very easy way to soften the wax is to cut a bit of the candle and place it into some hot water for a few minutes. Any method you want to use to soften the wax is fine. Put the piece of softened wax into the cavity and kind of smear it into place.

Gently bite down into the wax to make sure that your teeth come together properly. Slide the teeth back and forth a few times to be certain that your bite is correct. You'll know when that is. All your teeth will be contacting the way they were before you placed the temporary.

Avoid the area while eating and, when practical, call your dentist during his regular office hours. Don't awaken him for this one.

If there is no wax available, a piece of damp cotton will stay in the cavity reasonably well and will minimize that awful, cold sensitivity usually associated with a lost filling.

Lost Filling

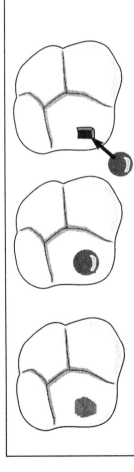

To temporarily replace a lost filling soften a bit of wax from a candle. (You can soften it by holding it in your hands or by putting it into hot water for a few minutes.) Smear the wax into the cavity so it fills the hole completely.

Bite down on the wax to make sure your bite is still the same as it was before you put the wax in. Scrape off the extra wax until your bite feels comfortable again. Get to your dentist soon, but you can wait until regular office hours for this one.

If you don't have any wax, some cotton will also work. You can also get material for a temporary filling at the pharmacy.

Do not place anything in a tooth that is throbbing or if there is any swelling. See the section on toothache instead.

You can purchase a more durable type of temporary filling if you go to the pharmacy. They are all non-prescription items and they are not too costly. Not a bad item to have around the house and in your travel kit, before the problem occurs.

Absolutely do *not* place any kind of temporary into a tooth that is throbbing or if there is any swelling in the area. If you are having these problems, go to page 34 (Toothache).

A lost filling is *not* a wake-your-dentist-up-at-midnight type of emergency, unless you don't particularly care for your dentist and you don't care what he thinks of you. I usually don't take sides, but in this instance I would side with the dentist. This is truly not an urgent situation. Call your dentist within the next couple of days or so, depending on how well you've made the temporary. On a quick five or ten minute appointment, he should be able to place a more secure temporary that will last until a more permanent procedure can be done.

By the way, regarding the wax, I strongly suggest that you not drip the wax directly from a lit candle into your mouth. Think it's a joke, huh?

I was called one evening by a patient who told me that a filling had dropped out and that the tooth was sensitive to cold. Over the phone, I explained how to use the wax properly. The patient was very thankful. I hung up after telling the patient to be at my doorstep the first thing in the morning. I thought I had temporarily relieved some discomfort and, at the same time, avoided my having to make an emergency trip to the office that evening.

The patient was waiting on my doorstep very early the next morning with one magnificent burn at the corner of his mouth. The wax temporary that he had placed was done very nicely, but this guy actually tried to drip the wax directly from the candle into his mouth. At least he started that way until he realized quite rapidly the error of his ways. I didn't tell him not to do it, did I? Was it his fault? My fault? Was he not thinking and did I just take something for granted?

Long story short, the burn healed, I fixed the tooth and all was wonderful again.

Stained or Discolored Teeth

People today are much more appearance conscious than in the past. This definitely includes, near the top of the list, concern about the appearance of their teeth. Cosmetic dentistry, because of this awareness, is rapidly evolving into a specialty field unto itself. Everybody wants to get into the act.

You have a variety of choices with stained or discolored teeth. Your choice will depend on the amount of staining and its cause and the amount you are willing to pay. So you ask: Cleaning? Bleaching? Veneers?

Twice-yearly visits to your dentist should include cleaning, scraping, scaling and polishing of your teeth. This professional cleaning should take care of most people's needs, as long as it is done regularly (and you don't smoke).

Bleaching, if it can be done, is the simplest and most effective treatment. It requires no grinding on the teeth and the outcome is fantastic. At least I had great results. I guess I was just a good operator (back pat). Usually bleaching is all the treatment you will require.

Veneers, both chairside and laboratory processed, are much more difficult than bleaching and are correspondingly more expensive. Both of these procedures, chairside and lab processed, will require that some grinding be done on the teeth. This grinding is superficial and might even be accomplished without the use of anesthetic (on you maybe, not on me).

With either bleaching or the application of veneers I have seen many people come out of their introverted shells when they are able to flash this new, dynamite smile. It can unquestionably create a new, more self-confident individual. To me, this was one of the more rewarding aspects of dentistry when I was in active practice.

Brushing or Professional Cleaning

If the problem is due to nothing more than food or tobacco stains and your regular toothpaste doesn't seem to clean properly, try brushing with a tooth powder or baking powder. They're a bit more abrasive than paste, but not abrasive enough to harm the teeth. As a matter of fact, either can be used routinely instead of your present paste. They're good. They do, however, lack fluoride. This is no real tragedy.

Proper brushing should take between three to five minutes. Anything less, you're doing yourself an injustice. If that doesn't work and the stains remain, see your dentist for a professional cleaning. It could be that the stain is adhering too firmly for simple brushing to remove completely. Professional cleaning should do the trick. Make certain that the teeth are scraped and scaled with those metal instruments that the dentist says you should never use to clean your teeth yourself. If only a simple polishing is done, they may not be doing a thorough job. Polishing is the *last* step done in a cleaning, not the only step.

Brushing Your Teeth

The purpose of brushing your teeth is to remove all of the stuff that gets stuck to them. It's called plaque. Leaving plaque on your teeth is a sure way to get gum disease and cavities.

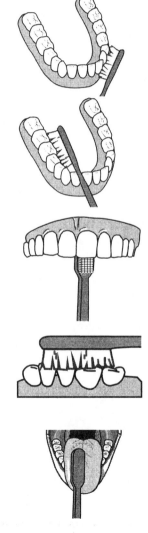

1. Start by brushing along the gum line using 1/4-inch strokes. The bristle tips should be pointed so they clean out the space between the gums and the teeth. Don't press too hard and let the bristle tips do the work.

2. Keep the bristles at the same angle and go over the surface of each tooth. Make sure to get both the outside and the inside with short, light strokes.

3. After you clean the outside of the front teeth be sure to get the inside, too, with the brush held in an almost vertical position. Use an up and down motion.

4. Clean the chewing surfaces of you molars and bicuspids. Take your time and get each tooth clean.

5. The final step is to brush your tongue. A few gentle strokes from back to front is sufficient. You don't have to brush back to your tonsils. Starting at about the midpoint is enough.

If the staining or discoloration is extreme and has been present for many years, it may be due to something other than food or tobacco. In these instances, neither bleaching nor meticulous professional cleaning will do the trick. I'll explain what might cause this type of staining when I discuss veneers on page 63.

Bleaching Your Teeth

I'm a firm believer in bleaching. It can truly cause a personality to bloom. It can create a radiant smile from what was once a half-hearted, dingy grin. This holds true for veneers as well. There are people who actually refuse to smile at all, only because they are ashamed of and embarrassed by the color of their teeth. They are not grouches, believe me. I am certain that they are experiencing feelings of extreme self-consciousness due to the discoloration of their teeth.

Bleaching Teeth

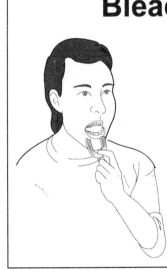

Moderate stains that have built up over the years can be often removed by bleaching. You can buy a do-it-yourself whitening kit or have it done professionally by your dentist. (The dentist costs more but should do a better job.)

A plastic appliance filled with bleaching gel is created to fit closely over the teeth. You wear it part of the time, usually at night, for two to four weeks.

If the darkening of your teeth is moderate and has gradually increased over the years, the bleaching procedure can definitely help. As individuals get older their teeth have a tendency to darken. This type of discoloration lends itself nicely to bleaching.

As much as I believe in bleaching, I'm also a firm advocate of saving money. If used properly, the do-it-yourself, home whitening kits that are sold over the counter are quite adequate. Follow directions carefully and the results can be gratifying. The cost can be in the vicinity of $40 to $60 for each arch. You will be using a technique and materials similar to what the dentist would use in his office.

The dentist, however, has in his office the proper materials and (hopefully) the proper skills to do the procedure more effectively than you will. The results will be correspondingly superior. The cost really isn't outrageous. Prices can range from $200 to $350 for each arch. The results are magic and are generally permanent. Some touchup in the future may be necessary, but it's a simple, painless procedure.

Professional bleaching is actually a very easy procedure. It does require a good deal of patient cooperation. A thin, clear, soft plastic appliance is made to fit closely over the teeth. A type of peroxide gel is squeezed into the plastic and then placed into the mouth. It must be worn for two to four weeks. It does not, however, have to be worn during the day. It can, in most instances, be worn each evening, while you are asleep. Some people prefer to wear the appliance during the day, which is fine. It's barely noticeable. Your speech may be a bit slurred initially, but after a few days you'll overcome that. If you wear it during the daytime, remove it while eating. You really don't want to chew it up. It's tasteless.

Have the upper arch completed first before having the lowers done. Many people will have just the uppers bleached as they only show their upper teeth when they talk and smile. This way, the cost of doing the lowers can be saved and used on something more enjoyable than the dentist.

Another logical reason to do one arch at a time is that you can truly see the contrast between the teeth that have been bleached and those that have not. If you like the results, you can then decide if you want to have the lowers done. If the results aren't what you expected, then you don't have to do the lowers.

Veneers

Veneers come into play when bleaching can't adequately do the job. If the discoloration is too severe, bleaching won't touch it. There are the unsightly, blotchy brown and chalky white discolorations that are likely caused by being exposed, as a child, to excessive amounts of fluoride in the drinking water. Similar deep staining might occur if large doses of tetracycline (an antibiotic) were taken in early childhood. This type of staining usually manifests itself as brownish or blue/purple bands traversing horizontally across the teeth. Both conditions will have been present since childhood. It's highly unlikely that stains of this nature would be correctable with professional bleaching. Veneers to the rescue.

There are techniques that your dentist can use to place veneers (false fronts) on the teeth very effectively. The cost per tooth depends on the technique that is used. Unfortunately, there are no home techniques for making veneers.

There are two basic types of veneers: chairside or laboratory processed.

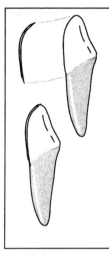

Veneers

Veneers can be used to cover discolored teeth that cannot be whitened by bleaching. Both chairside and laboratory veneers are available. Chairside veneers are faster and less expensive. Laboratory veneers are stronger and more lifelike. In both types of veneers a thin layer of material is bonded to the front of the tooth, hiding the discoloration.

Chairside veneers look good. These are veneers that the dentist places himself, without the assistance of a dental laboratory. A tooth-colored filling material is used that actually bonds to the front surface of your tooth. This procedure can be done in the office, quite possibly in just one visit. Since there are no lab fees involved, the cost is substantially less than with laboratory involvement. These restorations look good, are reasonably strong and function quite well.

Chairside veneers are much less expensive and take much less time. They can last anywhere from a year on up to four or five years, maybe more, depending on the patient's chewing habits and the dentist's expertise with the material. They are much easier to accomplish, both for the dentist and the patient, than are the laboratory veneers. They are also much more cost effective than their laboratory counterparts. Each chairside veneer can range anywhere between $135 to $250 per tooth.

Laboratory-processed veneers are better in all respects. They are veneers that are fabricated at a dental laboratory utilizing the joint skills of the dentist and the lab technician. They also are ultimately bonded to your teeth, as are the chairside restorations. A different, somewhat more powerful bonding technique is used, making these restorations much stronger than their chairside counterparts. Once bonded they wear like iron, yet in appearance they seem to be delicate, translucent and lifelike. This lab technique is far more difficult to do properly and requires at least two appointments.

Laboratory-processed veneers are much more expensive. If you can afford it, that's the path to take. Done properly, they are far more durable, substantially stronger and more pleasing in appearance than the chairside treatment. Cost per tooth can range anywhere between $400 to $800, depending on the rent that has to be paid by the dentist. The cost to you, the patient, is not the prime factor in determining the results. It's a combination of the expertise of the dentist, the lab and the materials used.

Don't get me wrong about chairside veneers. They are good and, if placed correctly using a sound technique and cared for properly, they can last a long time. I have placed many chairside veneers and a good portion of them have been in for well over five years and as far as I know are still functioning. Chairside veneers are also much easier and far less expensive to touch up if a chip occurs, than are the lab veneers.

I suppose it's kind of like the difference between a new VW and a new Mercedes. They are both new and they are both nice, but one is much nicer. Which one you buy is totally dependent on your bankroll. They both serve their purpose, don't they?

Chapter 4. Tissue

Teething

There is nothing more disturbing than to have your infant crying and your not being able to determine the cause. Maybe teething is the only problem. Baby teeth begin to erupt into the mouth when baby is somewhere between five and seven months old. If the baby is cranky for no apparent reason around this age, after you check for dirty diapers and all that good stuff, check the mouth. When teething occurs, the gums, usually in the lower front of the mouth, will be very swollen, sore and red. There will also be a ton of drooling. Baby is not a happy camper. Mommy and daddy are not happy either, because they are losing sleep, as well as losing their minds. The swelling, as a rule, starts in the lower gums, as the lower front baby teeth are typically the first to erupt. When the gums are rubbed lightly (if baby allows it),

---

Teething

The indications for teething are very swollen, sore and red gums and tons of drool. You may also be able to rub the gum lightly to see if you feel a sharp point. That's the new tooth coming in.

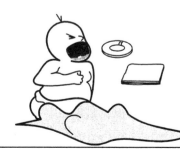 Some of the things that help relieve teething pain are a chilled (not frozen) teething ring and a chilled washcloth. Your baby can suck on those. You can also gently rub on any of the commercial teething medicines that contain benzocaine.

you may feel a sharp point. This is the new tooth poking its way into the mouth. It is the key to diagnosing the problem.

Chilled, gel-type teething rings — cold, but not frozen — are very effective in reducing the discomfort. Almost as effective, if the teething rings are not readily available, is to moisten a plain white washcloth with cold water. *Don't freeze it.* The baby can suck on the cloth for relief and you can gently pat, not rub, the gums with the cloth.

There are commercial products on the market for the relief of teething pain. They are all pretty good and are all about the same in terms of effectiveness. Almost each and every one contains a topical anesthetic called benzocaine that, when gently rubbed on the baby's gums, will numb the areas involved. These products, however, are never in your medicine cabinet at the right time. The cold wet cloth or the teething ring will do quite an effective job and they are cheaper.

Baby Tylenol or baby aspirin, with the pediatrician's approval, will very definitely help the baby and you to get some restful sleep, at least until baby is hungry again.

Teething, by the way, should not cause a fever. That's an old wives' tale. Fever means exactly what it indicates with everyone, infants and adults alike. It is an indication that an infection of some type is probably going on somewhere. If there is fever, contact your pediatrician. Teething causes irritation and inflammation to the gums, not infection.

Bleeding Gums

This section is very important because you could have problems. Please read it thoroughly.

Did you know that gum disease, not cavities, is far and away the leading cause of tooth loss in the adult population?

Home treatment is easy and can minimize the inflammation, but be aware that routine bleeding from the gums is not normal. It is typically caused by a soft bacterial plaque buildup at the base of the teeth. When not properly cleaned, this soft accumulation hardens and calcifies. This is commonly called tartar or calculus. This condition, when just starting, is referred to as gingivitis, which is nothing more than a fancy name for irritated, bleeding gums, and can quite readily be reversed. If left unattended, however, it can lead to more severe problems in the mouth. It is a warning. It's the old "teeth are good but the gums gotta go" syndrome. Only here, it could be gums, teeth and bone that might have to go.

If you're the type of person who routinely visits the dentist for cleanings and checkups, it may just be a matter of getting in for a simple cleaning and that's that. No big deal. Do it yesterday.

If you're the type who goes to the dentist, clawing and scratching, only when it's absolutely necessary, this gum condition could be the beginning and possibly the continuation of a very serious problem. Gum disease is a slowly blossoming entity that can go unnoticed day by day. Nevertheless, gradually and surely, it destroys the supporting structures surrounding the teeth.

If the bleeding and soreness are confined to only one area, you could be lucky. It might be nothing more than a localized traumatic irritation, possibly caused by jabbing yourself with a toothpick or a fork. You've really got to be clumsy to accomplish this, but it is a possibility.

Isolated irritation can also be caused by a particle of food or a foreign object that has wedged itself between the teeth. This annoyance is transient, and the irritation will be eliminated when the object is removed. The technique to remove objects is described on page 54 of this book. No treatment, other than rinsing, is necessary. However, if there is any doubt at all, you must see the dentist. You just can't get away from him/her, can you?

If the bleeding and/or soreness is generalized, extending over a number of areas, you absolutely must visit your dentist. Sorry about that, but this bleeding might even be a symptom of other general health problems. The important thing to realize is that any continual bleeding from the gums or, for that matter, from anywhere in the mouth, is *not normal* and should be treated accordingly.

The buildup of plaque and tartar (calcified garbage) sticks to the teeth, kind of like the way barnacles stick to the hull of a ship and like mussels to the pylons of a pier. It first starts to adhere to those parts of the teeth that are visible in the mouth. Then it continues to build up and work its way under the gums. The tartar is razor sharp. When any pressure is applied (such as with a toothbrush), the tartar is pushed against the gum tissue, causing tiny cuts and lacerations. It's this mechanical irritation that promotes the bleeding and the associated pain.

Brushing the teeth becomes a painful experience. The discomfort causes you to stay away from the areas involved. The brushing stops, allowing more tartar to accumulate and cause more pain and damage, creating a vicious circle.

Bleeding Gums and Gum Disease

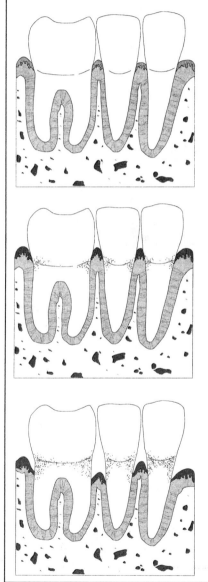

Bleeding gums are not normal. If the bleeding lasts more than a few days or occurs in several areas of the mouth, you must see your dentist. It certainly is a threat to your teeth and may be a symptom of other general health problems

Gum disease starts when plaque and tartar build up where the teeth and gums meet. Tartar is razor sharp and makes lots of little cuts in the gum tissue every time you eat or brush your teeth. The gums recede and the bone starts to recede, too, from the continued irritation. At some point there isn't enough bone to hold the teeth in place.

Go see your dentist early in the process and he can clean your teeth. That's all it takes early on. If you wait until you have advanced gum disease (periodontitus), you're looking at expensive and painful procedures.

This razor-sharp junk, if not professionally removed, actually travels down the root surface of the tooth, building up over a period of time. The accumulation will destroy the bone that supports the teeth. By the way, routine professional cleanings will virtually eliminate tartar buildup.

Visualize, if you will, a frying pan. The pan itself represents the body of your tooth, while the handle represents the root. Your hand, which will be gripping the handle, depicts the supporting bone. The heat generated from a nice hot flame will play the part of the tartar.

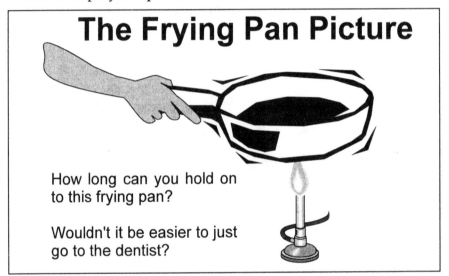

The Frying Pan Picture

How long can you hold on to this frying pan?

Wouldn't it be easier to just go to the dentist?

Envision the flame being placed under the cool pan. As the flame heats the pan, that heat travels from the pan to its handle, the root of the tooth. Your hand, the bone, begins to feel the heat and moves backwards on the handle until it can't tolerate the heat any longer. Your hand ultimately has to let go and the pan, your tooth, falls out. Get it?

The condition, when it reaches this stage, is called advanced periodontitis and advanced gum disease. Sorry to throw some of these technical terms at you.

Just remember, gingivitis can be the beginning of perio-dontitis and periodontitis can be the end of your teeth. My lecture on this subject is over. See your dentist routinely and it won't happen.

Bleeding, Inflamed Gums (Gingivitis)

For both generalized and local inflammation, use warm salt water or a mixture with equal amounts of warm water and hydrogen peroxide solution. Rinse vigorously as needed. I mean *really* squish that water through and between the teeth. When you brush the teeth, don't avoid the areas that are sore. Just brush a bit more gently, but do brush them. You can bet the mortgage that the gums will bubble and bleed, but this bleeding, believe it or not, can be benefi-cial in that it may help to wash out any loose foreign parti-cles from around and beneath the gums. As I said before, go see your dentist, too.

Bleeding in and around the Mouth and Lips (Usually Trauma Induced)

Take a washcloth dampened with cold water and hold it directly over the injured area, using moderate, steady pres-sure to control the bleeding. If a youngster is involved, a red or black cloth would be nice as it will mask the color of the blood and minimize the emotional stress to all concerned (especially the parent). Almost always the bleeding will stop. Give it a few minutes.

If the bleeding doesn't stop after a few minutes or if there is spurting blood, keep pressure on the area to slow the bleeding as much as possible and go to an emergency care location immediately.

Bleeding from an Injury

Keep calm.

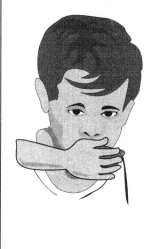

Take a washcloth dampened with cold water and hold it directly over the injured area. Using a black or red washcloth will mask the blood and make you feel better. It might even be easier for the person who got hurt.

Hold the cloth on with moderate pressure until the bleeding stops. It may take a few minutes. If the bleeding doesn't stop in a few minutes or there is spurting blood, keep pressure on and go to an emergency room right away.

After the bleeding stops, continue the pressure for a few more minutes. Then switch to an ice pack to reduce the swelling. Don't leave it on for more than 15 minutes at a time.

When the bleeding is controlled, continue the moderate pressure for a few more minutes, then switch to an ice pack. A frozen juice can or a bag of frozen vegetables wrapped in a towel will do nicely. This will keep the swelling to a minimum. Don't forget, when using the ice pack, do not keep it on the area for more than ten to fifteen minutes at a time, followed by ten to fifteen minutes off.

When the lips and/or the gums are lacerated and bleeding, the lip(s) will swell considerably, regardless of the ice pack application. Looks awful. Believe me, it almost always looks much worse than it really is. The cold washcloth, along with the ice packs, will reduce the swelling and help to numb the area, keeping the discomfort down. The moderate pressure will help control the bleeding.

If there's only a small laceration, stitches probably won't be necessary. The smallest cuts in or around the lips and mouth will seem much worse because the lips and mouth have an abundant blood supply and tend to bleed rather heavily when injured. The fact that there is lots of blood in the area is also the primary reason that mouth wounds heal rapidly.

Keep calm and, if a child is involved, don't show any undue fright on your part.

Excessive Bleeding after an Extraction

As Murphy's Law goes, your dentist takes off for a golf game 30 minutes after he extracts your tooth and forgets to take his beeper. Now your gum is bleeding at the extraction site and you can't reach your dentist. So what do you do? A small amount of bleeding and oozing, for about twenty-four hours after an extraction, is normal. The saliva might be tinged with a pinkish color. It's human nature for the tongue to get nosey and start playing with the space where the tooth used to be. This can cause some additional bleeding, so keep your tongue away and don't play.

If you are not allergic to tea, moisten a teabag and place it in your mouth over the extraction area. Bite down with moderate pressure for about a half an hour. This should minimize, if not totally stop, the bleeding. (Use either black or green tea that contains tannins. Not all herbal teas do.)

You may repeat this procedure a few times if necessary, each time using a new tea bag. Do not rinse your mouth directly over the extraction area for a period of twenty-four hours as you may wash away the forming blood clot. This can create a rather painful condition called "dry socket," which usually requires another trip (oh, God, no) to the dentist.

If heavy, bright red bleeding persists and can't be controlled, contact your dentist as soon as possible. There is probably something in the socket causing the bleeding. In some instances it's nothing more than a loose piece of bone that's rubbing against the gums and the dentist can just pluck it out, hopefully at no additional charge. Complain loudly if there is a charge. Naturally, wait until he's finished with the procedure before you yell. Don't want an angry dentist working on your mouth, do you? You may need to consider going to your local emergency room if your dentist cannot be reached. Then try to find another family dentist who is more readily available.

Pain and Swelling after an Extraction

To control the pain, usually the dentist will choose to prescribe some type of pain medication to carry you through the worst of it. If not, just ask him for something. "The squeaky wheel gets greased." Beg if you must.

Most pain killers are very effective in controlling post-extraction pain. If the dentist doesn't think you'll need anything for the pain, he could be right. But he could also be wrong. Many easy extractions don't require any medication at all. If he's wrong and you can't reach him to call in a prescription for you, after you cuss him out, take some acetaminophen (Tylenol) or ibuprofen (Advil). Both work admirably and neither requires a prescription.

Do not take aspirin. Even though aspirin is generally a wonder drug, it can cause problems if taken after an extraction. It promotes bleeding and slows down the clotting process considerably. Don't use it after extractions. Okay?

Pain after an Extraction

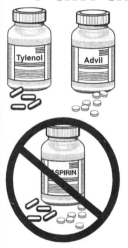

Usually your dentist will give you a perscription to get you through the worst of the post-extraction pain. You can even ask him for one. If he doesn't give you a prescription and the extraction site really hurts, you will probably get plenty of relief from Tylenol (acetaminophen) or Advil (ibuprofin). Don't take aspirin, though. It will make the bleeding worse. Ice packs help, too. Don't leave them on for more than 20 minutes at a time.

To control swelling, as well as pain, ice the area for the first twenty-four hours. A good ice pack can be made by wrapping a frozen juice can or a bag of frozen vegetables in a towel. Place it externally over the extraction site.

Keep it on for about fifteen to twenty minutes, then off for about the same period of time. This can be done a number of times during the first 24 hours after extraction. Then, on the day after the extraction, after a full 24 hours, switch to heat, using warm salt water rinses. Be very gentle. If you are too vigorous about rinsing, you might wash out the blood clot. This can lead to a rather painful complication.

In most cases the pain after an extraction will not be too bad, as long as it happens to you and not to me. It will subside gradually within a period of a few days. If the pain intensifies and hangs around for more than a few days, it would be wise to call your dentist. It well might be an indication of a beginning problem that should be treated with medication. Usually the pain associated with an extraction is directly related to the time and difficulty involved in removing the tooth, more the difficulty than the time.

It reminds me of the story of the patient who went to see the dentist with a wracking toothache. The dentist saw the patient immediately and with skilled hands removed the culprit tooth with minimal discomfort to the patient and in record time. The patient was out of the dental chair in a matter of minutes.

When asked, "How much?" the dentist replied, "That will be $100." The patient's eyes opened wide and he was visibly very upset. "Hey, doc, that's an awful lot of money for such a short period of time. Isn't there anything you can do?" the patient asked. The dentist, without hesitation, responded, "Yes, there is. Next time I can pull the tooth v-e-r-y s-l-o-w-l-y." The patient paid without further comment.

Canker Sores

Canker sores appear as small ulcerations, usually circular or oval in shape, with a yellowish-white center, surrounded by an inflamed red ring. The ulcers usually appear on, around and under the tongue and anywhere on the gums and inside the cheeks. They are extremely sore and sensitive to the touch.

The key is to reduce the duration, which is about seven to ten days, and hopefully reduce the discomfort associated with the sores.

A mixture with equal amounts of warm water and hydrogen peroxide solution is beneficial. This is to be swished around in the mouth over the affected areas and then rinsed out, not swallowed. Do this as frequently as you wish. Eight to ten times each day is fine.

The use of Orabase or Orabase B, the mouth bandage, can be helpful in covering the ulcers and protecting them from further irritation. You can buy these in the pharmacy. Follow product instructions. They works well.

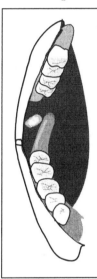

Canker Sores

Canker sores are small circular or oval ulcerations with a yellowish-white center surrounded by an inflamed red ring. They can appear anywhere inside the mouth: on the tongue, under the tongue, on the gums or inside the cheeks.

One thing that helps is swishing the mouth with a solution of half water and half hydrogen peroxide solution. You can also apply ice, Orabase (or Orabase B) or teabags to the affected area.

Place a teabag on the affected area for about ten to twenty minutes. It will help to minimize the discomfort. (Use teabags that contain tannic acid such as black tea.) This can be done a few times each day.

Ice applied directly to the area can help diminish the irritation. Remember, don't keep it on the area too long.

Common sense dictates that you stay away from spicy foods. They will further inflame the ulcers.

To date, no one knows what causes these miserable things. The sores may be a reaction to certain bacteria, or they could be trauma (injury) related, such as jabbing yourself with the butt end of a toothbrush. Don't tell me that you have never done that. Stress also could be a causative factor. One positive note is that these ulcers usually heal spontaneously, whether treated or not. Unless they are rampant and frequent, no prescription medication is necessary. If they are more than an infrequent nuisance, your physician or dentist can prescribe a medicated mouthwash.

Canker sores occur most frequently inside the mouth, while fever blisters/cold sores (Herpes) will occur primarily outside the mouth, around the red border of the lips.

Cold Sores/Fever Blisters (Herpes)

The symptoms of cold sores are a tingling, burning sensation around the lips, with small, clear, fluid-filled blisters arranged in grape-like clusters, usually on or near the lips, itching like mad.

If the sores are minor and occur infrequently, they will run their course of about seven to ten days and that will be that. If they are severe, there are several things that can be done to reduce the discomfort and hasten the healing. There are also treatments that can minimize their recurrence.

If you're planning to be out in the sun, use sunscreen as a preventative measure.

Apply ice to the affected area. This can reduce the discomfort and possibly hasten the healing process. Place the ice in a zip lock bag. Wrap it in a thin towel and don't keep it on the area for more than ten minutes at a time.

Cold Sores

Cold sores start with a tingling, burning sensation around the edges of the lips. The sensation is followed by small, clear, fluid-filled blisters arranged in clusters. They itch like crazy.

It's very important not to get any of the fluid from the blisters on anyone else. The herpes virus that causes the cold sores can be transmitted to others. Kissing, unfortunately, is out until the blisters heal. Ice will help relieve the itching.

Go to the dietary supplement section of your pharmacy and you will find a product called Lysine. This may be used routinely as a dietary supplement and it can help reduce the recurrence and the severity of the sores. Purchase the 500 mg. tablets. You can take up to three tablets each day, one in the morning, one in the afternoon and one at night. They are very reasonably priced, if in fact any item in the pharmacy can be considered as reasonably priced.

There is also a prescription drug available that is effective if your problem is severe. The drug is called Acyclovir, brand name, Zovirax. It comes in either ointment or capsule form. Check with your physician or dentist as to which he thinks will best suit your needs. Both require a prescription. Long term treatment with the capsules can be very successful in drastically reducing, if not eliminating, the return of the virus. I hope you've got insurance. The capsules cost a bundle.

Once you've got fever blisters, you've got 'em for life. These blisters are caused by the herpes simplex virus. The virus can, and usually does, lie dormant in your system for years. It becomes active during periods of stress, localized irritation and lowered resistance. Exposure to sunlight and wind, both being irritants, can initiate an outbreak.

During an acute episode, cleanliness is very important. When these blisters are "weeping," they can be transmitted to others, causing them to be infected also. You can wave hello or goodbye to your love, just don't kiss. Sorry about that, but don't feel too bad. If misery loves company, a good percentage of the population has these things. Mostly they are embarrassing and annoying, nothing more, nothing less.

Sore Spots on Gums from Denture Rubbing

If sores are an uncommon occurrence, happening maybe once every six to eight months, and they heal rapidly, it's probably nothing more than a seed or some other piece of junk lodged underneath the denture, next to the gums. This can be an exquisite source of pain.

Fortunately, almost immediately after the culprit is removed, the irritation heals. Other than some warm salt water rinses to help pull out any remaining irritation, no treatment is necessary. Cost to you, $0.00.

If a sore starts and the warm salt water doesn't correct the problem after a day or so, there are a couple of other things that you can try in an attempt to ease the discomfort.

Get an indelible pencil and dull the point. If the point is not dulled, you'll almost certainly stab yourself and tattoo the spot in the mouth that you've just poked with the sharp pencil. So, please, dull the tip. Then take the denture out of your mouth and set it aside, nearby. Find the sore spot in your mouth by touching it with your fingertip. Then touch it a few times with the indelible pencil.

Sore Spots from Dentures

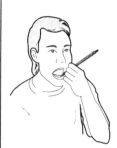

Small bumps on the insides of dentures can cause continuing irritation to your gums. To find the spot that is causing the trouble, get an indelible pencil and dull the point. Find the sore spot in your mouth by touching it with your finger tip. Then touch the same spot a few times with the indelible pencil.

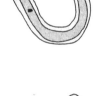

Place the denture back in your mouth and bite down to the point of discomfort. Hold the teeth together for a few seconds and then take the denture out of your mouth again.

You should see a blue mark on the inside of the denture. It marks the spot that is bothering you. If you are adventurous, you can use an emery board (the fine side) to scrape some of the plastic away. Ten to twenty strokes should do it. Rinse the denture and see if the "ouch" is gone. If not, you can take a little more plastic off.

If you don't want to scrape your denture, a wisp of damp cotton on the mark will ease the pain until you get to the dentist.

There are some adjustments that you can't make yourself. If you have continuing problems or a sore that doesn't seem to heal, go see your dentist right away.

This will leave a temporary mark on the gums. It might be a tad uncomfortable, but that's an indication that you're right on the money, hitting the irritated area. Don't bother looking in your mouth for the mark. Trust me on this one. It'll be there.

Then place the denture back into your mouth and bite down to the point of discomfort. Who are we kidding? Bite or tap the teeth together until you feel the pain. Maintain some pressure for a few seconds and then take the denture out of your mouth again. You should have a nice dark blue mark on the inside of the denture, transferred from the spot where it was rubbing in your mouth. If the marking isn't there, no big deal. Just repeat the procedure.

Take an emery board and use the fine side. Rub it back and forth over the blue spot, including a small area outside the spot. You will see some of the plastic being scraped away. Apply moderate pressure while you rub, for about ten to twenty strokes. Then rinse the denture and put it back in. The acute soreness should be gone. Some soreness will still be present since the area has already been irritated and might be a bit swollen. The sharp "ouch," however, should be gone. If it isn't, go ahead and use the emery board again. You probably didn't take enough off. If this works as planned, you may not even have to see the dentist.

If you're not adventurous and don't want to try scraping away any plastic, if all you want is some relief until you can reach your dentist, here's what to do, you coward.

Simply take a wisp of cotton, moisten it and place it in the denture directly over the corresponding sore spot in your mouth. This will raise the denture off the irritated area and will afford you some relief. You can moisten the cotton with any teething medicine that has Benzocaine (a topical anesthetic) in it. This will numb the area. Then see your dentist and he will be able to trim the spot for you.

If you are having continual problems with denture sores and you have the same sore that doesn't seem to heal completely, it still may be only an adjustment of the denture that you can't accomplish adequately yourself. It may be that you need a reline (which I explain on page 106) or it may be something more serious. Suffice it to say that chronic, frequent soreness is not normal and must be treated professionally. Don't procrastinate.

Burns Inside Mouth Because of Hot Food/Drinks

Very easy. Use ice water or a cold soda, the sooner, the better. The ice will immediately reduce the pain and will minimize the tissue reaction.

To promote healing and to soothe the tissue when you get home, continue with the iced drinks to help reduce any swelling and to numb the area. The following day start rinsing gently with a half teaspoon of delicious table salt dissolved in a glass of warm water. Rinse four or five times daily for a couple of days and the area will heal quite rapidly. If the burn is really uncomfortable, go to the dental health section of your pharmacy and pick up some Orabase, the mouth bandage that actually sticks to the moist gums. This will help to protect the burn from further irritation. Orabase B is the same product with a topical anesthetic included in its formula.

Regardless of whether the area is treated or not, the tissue will heal. It will do so even without treatment, more slowly perhaps, but it will heal. The recuperative capabilities of mouth tissue are incredible.

Burns in the Mouth

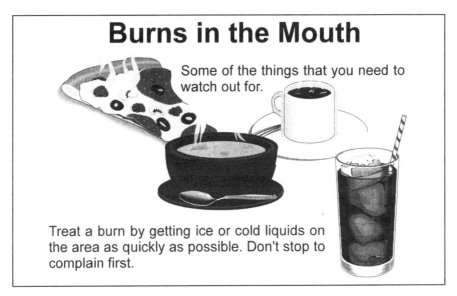

Some of the things that you need to watch out for.

Treat a burn by getting ice or cold liquids on the area as quickly as possible. Don't stop to complain first.

It might be worthwhile to talk briefly about prevention. I'll bet you've burned your mouth more than once on pizza. Haven't you ever stuffed that first piece of pizza, with all that delicious sizzling cheese on it, into your mouth minutes after the pizza is out of the oven? I have, more than once. I guess I never learn. It almost inevitably finds its way to the roof of the mouth directly behind the front teeth and it sticks there like hot tar. It's only funny when it happens to someone else.

It will probably cause some minor damage to the palatal tissue located right behind the upper front teeth, just because you weren't fast enough with the ice. As you probably noticed, putting ice on the area is not the first thing that people do. First they make noises, then they say some things that are not so nice and then, finally, the ice goes to the area. You could, of course, do the logical thing and wait until the food cools a bit before you eat, but that's unrealistic, especially with pizza, isn't it?

No other comments. We really don't deserve any sympathy, do we? All we have to do is to wait a couple of minutes for the food to cool and it won't happen. Right? Your palate will thank you.

Tongue or Cheek Biting

Who in this world has never bitten his tongue or cheek? Maybe that should be rephrased to read: How many times have you bitten yourself this month?

For the most part, there is no remedy for tongue or cheek biting. It's a self-imposed, self-limiting, cuss-word-evoking incident that will cause a good deal of discomfort (especially the next day, when you bite the same place again) and bleeding.

The discomfort might be temporarily minimized with the use of some type of topical numbing agent. Regardless of what is done, however, that raw tissue will be with you, extremely sensitive and prone to re-injury until it heals.

If this is a continual problem, it could be that the teeth don't come together properly, creating premature contacting of certain teeth. This sometimes occurs after a new bridge or denture is placed and can be corrected by the dentist with some rounding over of the culprit tooth or teeth on the bridge so that they don't hit the opposing teeth too soon.

Overweight people, with chubby cheeks, are more prone to cheek biting than thinner people.

Chapter 5: Braces

Orthodontics

Orthodontics is that dental specialty dealing with the correction of poorly positioned teeth in an attempt to maximize function and appearance. It is usually not started until most, if not all, of the permanent teeth have erupted. Some interceptive (preventative) orthodontics is done earlier, attempting to simplify and minimize the corrective phase of treatment.

There are basically two types of orthodontic appliances.

Removable appliances that are used when there is mild-to-moderate correction necessary, usually involving minor movement of only a few teeth.

Fixed appliances (cemented or bonded) that are used when the case is more difficult, requiring movement of a number of teeth. This type of treatment gives rise to the classic railroad track appearance of the mouth (braces).

Brackets are bonded to the teeth and a continuous wire band is slipped through openings in the brackets. Tension on the wire is adjusted to facilitate tooth movement.

Teens don't really rebel at the prospect of wearing braces. It's kind of a status symbol. Further, being very concerned with appearance, they realize that future improvement in looks will follow treatment.

One of the major problems with orthodontics is that meticulous care must be given to the teeth. Braces create nooks and crannies where food particles can kick back, relax, hide and rot. This hidden rubbish can be secure in the knowledge that it will be difficult to locate, kind of like a criminal having established the ultimate hideout.

I mentioned previously that teens have the highest decay rate of all the age groups. This, combined with placement of orthodontic braces, requires continual professional and parental nagging. Laying guilt trips regarding cost of treatment is well within legal limits. Anything that works is acceptable. Proper brushing is essential, at least twice daily.

Braces

Braces are almost a rite of passage for teens. If your teen is "blessed" with the chance to wear braces, prepare to nag, complain, lecture and threaten to make sure that your child takes proper care of his or her teeth. There are so many places that nasty, decay-causing food particles can hide.

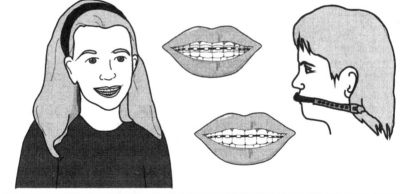

Regular dental checkups and cleanings are of utmost importance, *especially* when orthodontia is being accomplished. With orthodontic braces in position, it is difficult at best for the dentist to examine all the tooth surfaces thoroughly, even with x-rays. You can begin to see the importance of the home care, of the exams, of the fluoride, of the nagging and of my lecturing (which I despise, but I do).

Flossing is only minimally beneficial in a fully banded mouth. The floss can't effectively be snapped down between the teeth to the gum line because of the continuous arch wire threaded through the braces. You must approach the gum line from beneath the braces. I suggest, as an adjunct to brushing, using the Water Pik (page 129) and Stimudents (page 54).

One last thought on orthodontics. Many orthodontists are in the habit of recycling brackets for re-use. They are fully sterilized and used again on different patients. This is primarily done for economic reasons. New brackets cost the orthodontist somewhere between three and four dollars each. If recycled, the cost drops to about thirty cents apiece. This can amount to savings for the practitioner of seventy to one hundred dollars each mouth. In a large, clinic-type practice, that could amount to a substantial overhead reduction.

Parents might consider asking the orthodontist if new or recycled brackets are being used, so as to have the savings passed on. Others might not like the idea of something that was previously used in another mouth being placed in their child's mouth. If that's the case, simply ask for new. There's a mild controversy going on about this practice with the brackets. I won't get involved.

All four of my kids wore braces. Personally I didn't care whether the brackets were recycled or new, as long as proper sterilization methods were used and as long as the results were not compromised. Besides, treatment was done on my three older kids by a very dear friend and the price was right. A similar situation existed for my younger son. I didn't complain, but I'm not you.

Adult Orthodontics

In today's society, obsessed with appearance, straightening of adult teeth is becoming increasingly popular. Moving adult teeth is somewhat more difficult than moving a teenager's teeth. Growth patterns in the mouth stop in the late teens. The bone becomes denser and the teeth, therefore, become harder to move. (Is this why adults are considered hard headed?)

Orthodontics works basically on two principles, the controlled destruction of bone and its regeneration. Bone is being broken down as the tooth is being moved and regenerates when it is being stabilized. Bone regeneration occurs more rapidly for youngsters, so the teeth can be moved faster, but not too fast. Haste makes waste. Moving teeth too quickly will create problems.

Extra care must be taken with adults. Movement must be slower as regeneration is slower. If teeth are moved too hastily, bone destruction will occur more swiftly than regeneration, causing stability problems and, at its worst, tooth loss. Any competent orthodontist knows this and will be able to cope with the impatient patient.

Orthodontic Wires or Bands Cutting into the Gums

If your child and, for that matter, if you are having some tooth straightening done, you should always have a bit of beeswax available. It can be purchased at the pharmacy or it may be given to you by the orthodontist. Just ask him or her. You can just roll some of the wax into a little ball about the size of a pea and push it over the sharp edge of the wire or band that is cutting the gums or the cheek. This will handle the problem until you can see the orthodontist.

Problems with Wires

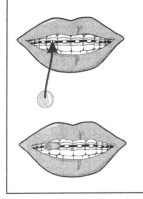

The wires or bands on a set of braces can sometimes cut into the gums. To solve the problem until you can see your dentist, take a small ball of beeswax and push it on the sharp edge of the wire or band. Go see your orthodontist. It should be taken care of free of charge.

He'll just bend or smooth the wire or band that's causing the irritation and that'll be that. No pain, no fuss, no bother, no charge. There shouldn't be any charge; he's getting enough from you as it is.

If the wire or a band has broken, a new one will be made. Again, it really should be at no charge.

If beeswax is not available, simply place a small piece of cotton over the sharp edge. You can moisten the cotton, if you like, with some teething medicine to numb the irritated area. You can also use Orabase B on the irritated area. This is the "oral bandage" that contains a topical anesthetic. It can be purchased at any pharmacy.

This was really so simple I was hesitant to write about it. Yet I couldn't leave it out because it does occur rather frequently and if there just happened to be one person who didn't know about the simplicity of this treatment, then I've helped someone, haven't I?

For instance, what if it's on a weekend and you can't reach the orthodontist because he doesn't carry his cellular phone with him on the golf course. Even if he did carry it, he wouldn't pick up because he knows that it's you calling.

Now you don't even need him. You can temporarily correct the situation yourself. You can both cover the sharp point and numb the area. This can all be done while the dentist finishes his round of golf. Then, bill him for your services.

Good luck.

Orthodontic Bands

The experience my kids had with their ortho bands was, for the most part, relatively easy. Actually, the bands were tooth savers in one particular instance.

When he was about fourteen years old, my older boy was in full orthodontic bands and just happened one day to run into a fist (naturally, through no fault of his own).

By virtue of these well-placed knuckles, his two upper front teeth were pushed upwards and backwards at least a good half inch. Had it not been for the banding, the teeth would have been completely knocked out.

One of my close friends was an orthodontist so I immediately took my son to his office (didn't even have an appointment). We gave my son a local anesthetic to minimize the discomfort. We then repositioned the teeth (forcefully pushed them back into place) and re-banded them. This was about fifteen years ago. The teeth are still there, in good alignment, and are quite solid.

My other son's karate lessons bother me though.

Chapter 6: Dentures

Think about this. If you don't have dentures, stick two chunks of square plastic, about three inches by three inches by one inch in your mouth. Then try to talk or, better yet, try to eat something. That'll give you some idea as to how dentures might feel in your mouth. I sincerely hope you never have to experience them. It just isn't fun. At best they are tolerable substitutes for your natural teeth.

If reality is upon you and your choice is between having to wear dentures and gumming your food, read the following. It may help you to understand what you can expect from your dentures.

Ideally, if you must have dentures, you should have two sets made. A spare set of dentures can eliminate some seriously awkward moments, especially if your upper denture is chewed up by the dog or sneezed out the car window while you're doing seventy on the freeway. Being without the lower isn't quite as bad, appearance wise, but it's bad enough. If you aren't fortunate enough ($$$$$) to have two sets of dentures made, then just be very aware of that fact and treat your dentures accordingly.

Dentures: The Graveyard of Dentistry

Have you heard this one?

"Get your teeth pulled and your problems will be over!" Trust me on this one. Your troubles will just be starting. Your steaks may have to be put in the blender. Your ice cube crunching days may be over and your sensation of taste will be drastically reduced. Granted, there are exceptions to every rule. There are denture wearers that truly swear *by* their false teeth. Most people, however, swear *at* them, continually. They are tolerated at best, because there are few other options available.

There are specialists who make implants. This is a relatively new procedure whereby dentures are kind of screwed into the bone. When they work, they're great. They are very costly, difficult to do, and upkeep on the patient's part is quite extensive.

The more normal, removable false teeth require quite a bit of care themselves. They must be brushed and cleaned to keep them sanitary and fresh. Bacteria and tartar can develop on dentures just as they can on natural teeth. Fortunately the denture teeth won't rot, but they sure will stain and stink.

I've seen dentures so loaded with tartar, it would take a crowbar and a day and a half to properly clean them. Not only is this unsightly, but it's an unhealthy condition. In addition to the necessity of dentures having to be brushed daily, they should be soaked frequently in any commercial denture-cleaning solution (follow product instructions). Special brushes and pastes are available specifically for these appliances. *Denture-cleansing pastes are far too abrasive for natural teeth and should be used only on dentures.*

Denture Tooth Falling Out

You just might be able to fix this yourself as a reasonably permanent repair. It may end up being temporary but, if a front tooth comes off a denture, temporary is much better than nothing.

Here's a technique that holds true for both the front and back teeth: Super Glue it.

But wait a minute. Isn't Super Glue poisonous? Should it be used in the mouth? Let me answer these questions by asking a few other questions. Isn't fluoride a poison? Isn't chlorine a poison? Isn't mercury a poison?

The answer to all of these questions is a resounding, "YES!" In their pure form, if incorrectly used in *improper amounts*, all can be deadly. Yet fluoride and chlorine in drinking water (in their proper percentages) are not only safe, but are beneficial.

Mercury is used in the standard basic silver dental filling. Standing along, it is a poison, but when mixed in combination with silver, copper, tin and zinc, it becomes an inactive, very strong material that has been used to fill teeth almost since the beginning of modern dentistry.

Super Glue, when used properly, becomes, after it hardens, a solid, strong bonding agent very similar chemically to the bonding agents that are used to place the tooth-colored fillings now routinely used in dentistry.

The technique that I'm about to describe is done completely outside the mouth. The repair is not placed into the mouth until it is completed and the material is hardened. It *is* safe.

First, have some nail polish remover, some alcohol, a toothbrush and the glue available. When you have all these things right in front of you, then you can begin.

I'm assuming that you still have the tooth. If you don't and it happens to be a back tooth, no big deal. Just forget about it. If it's a front tooth and it can't be found, find the whitest candle you can locate, drip some wax into the area where the tooth was and try to carve something that resembles a tooth. Needless to say, you'll be at the dental office immediately.

If you do have the tooth, here's the technique. Clean the tooth and the pink plastic base of the denture, especially in the area where the tooth was located. First, use soap and water and scrub those areas. Then, use rubbing alcohol on the toothbrush and scrub again. When the tooth and the denture plastic are thoroughly clean, make sure that they are *totally dry*. Then (*and this is very important*) make certain that the tooth goes right back to its proper original position. There will be a semicircular depression or shelf or ledge in the pink plastic of the denture into which the bottom, non-biting end of the tooth, fits. It will almost "snap" into its correct location.

When you are as certain as you can be that the tooth is in its correct position in the denture plastic, remove it and do it again. You should do this two, three and four times in succession. Silly, you say? *I think not.* This repetition will give you the exact feel of the tooth when it is in its proper spot. This is of utmost importance. If you've ever used Super Glue before, no further explanation is required.

Place one drop of the glue, any brand will do, onto the pink denture base where the tooth fell out. Position the tooth exactly as you practiced before. There is no need to rush. Hold it steady for about thirty seconds or whatever time the glue instructions indicate. You don't have to apply a lot of pressure. Then, let the denture sit for about five minutes. Don't even think about touching the blessed thing. This should do it. This repair could hold anywhere from hours to days, weeks, months, years, etc. No telling. It will, with minimal care, certainly hold until you can get to the dentist.

Replacing a Denture Tooth

Remove the denture from your mouth.

Using a toothbrush, scrub the tooth and the denture with soap and water. Scrub it again with rubbing alcohol until it is thoroughly clean. Then make sure that it is *totally dry*.

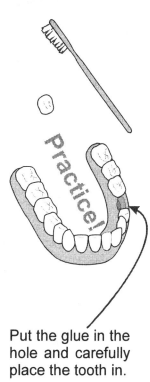

Put the tooth into the hole and make sure it fits properly. Do this three or four times to make sure that you know exactly how it fits. Super Glue does not give you a second chance.

If you're sure you want to try this, put a drop of glue onto the denture base where the tooth fell out. Position the tooth just like you practiced and hold it for thirty seconds or so. (Read the instructions on the glue.) Then let it sit for five minutes.

Put the glue in the hole and carefully place the tooth in.

If you position the tooth incorrectly, quickly wiggle it a few times and take it out. Use nail polish remover to dissolve the glue. Clean the area again with rubbing alcohol. Now you can try again.

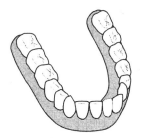

Now, *horror of horrors*, if you were clumsy and the tooth didn't go into place properly, all is not lost yet. Well, maybe not. Immediately take the tooth out. Wiggling the tooth forward and backward a few times will loosen the bond and you'll be able to remove it. A drop of the nail polish remover will help. Then scrub both the tooth and the "socket" area of the denture, only this time do it with nail polish remover on the toothbrush. The nail polish remover acts as a solvent for the glue. Thoroughly rinse both the tooth and the denture while scrubbing with the toothbrush. There will be an exam on this later.

Dry the areas again completely. Any moisture at all is death to the bonding power of the glue. Clean again with rubbing alcohol, dry again and try again. Go for it. The worst you can do is mess up the tooth. If your attempt at a repair is a complete failure and it doesn't work, so what. You have to get it fixed anyway. You really haven't lost anything. The professional repair will still cost about the same.

If the tooth is a plastic tooth, the repair will hold longer than for a porcelain tooth. How, you ask, can you tell which is plastic and which is porcelain? Do you really care? If the curiosity is killing you and you must put this tidbit of information in your book of useless knowledge, the *porcelain* front denture teeth have one or two small metal pins sticking out from the back side of the tooth that contacts the pink denture plastic. The *plastic* teeth don't have these pins. Isn't that fascinating?

Broken Denture Base

A *partial fracture* that hasn't completely broken through, or a chunk of the pink denture plastic that has broken out, doesn't really require instant attention. You don't have to drop everything and immediately run to the dentist. The partial fracture will probably appear to be a hairline, usually running from front to back. If that hairline goes all the way to the back of the plate, get to the dentist just a bit sooner than if the line doesn't go all the way back. Just be exceptionally careful and you should be able to wear the plate without any problem until a repair can be done.

Cracked Denture

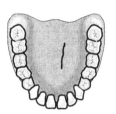

A cracked denture can be annoying but, luckily, it does not require instant attention. For a small hairline crack like the one in the top picture, you eventually need to get to the dentist and have it repaired. If you're careful, there is no real rush.

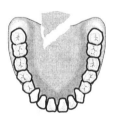

A plate with a crack that goes all the way to the back (second picture) is a little less sturdy so you should get to the dentist a little sooner.

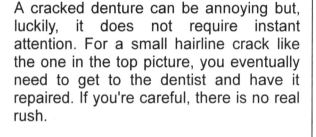

If a piece has broken out, as in the third picture, it really shouldn't cause you any trouble. You might try the repair yourself (see the text) or you can let your dentist handle it. Save the piece and take it with you to your dentist.

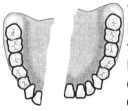

When you have a complete fracture, it's best to have it professionally repaired. In the meantime, use denture adhesive, a lot of denture adhesive, to keep the denture in place (and you smiling and eating) until you can get to the dentist and have it fixed.

With the partial fracture, the parts are not completely separated. Naturally, be rather cautious about biting too hard. This type of repair is a relatively simple one for the dentist and can probably be done while you wait and hide. You should get to your dentist as soon as it is practical. No emergency, but the longer you wait, the greater the chance of the break's becoming larger and ultimately splitting in two or more pieces. This will create a more difficult repair.

If it's a chunk of the plastic that has broken away, you can, if you like, attempt to Super Glue the chunk back into place, using the same technique as just described for the tooth (page 99). Just make certain that the parts oppose properly and go into place easily.

If you choose not to try the repair, save the piece. You should still be able to function with your denture nicely. If you don't see any other "hairlines" in the denture caused by your clumsiness, this type of repair can wait until it's convenient for you to get to the office. The dentist should be able to get this repaired in quick order and the plate will be as good as new.

A *complete fracture* through the upper denture, more often than not, will occur from front to back. A complete fracture of the lower denture, usually happens in the front segment, between the lower front teeth. These breaks are usually in two and, at worst, in three large pieces.

These fractures can be handled by you very simply and effectively. Regardless of how you handle it, however, you must ultimately have a professional repair done. This is strictly temporary.

Use some denture adhesive. Actually use *a lot* of denture adhesive. Don't worry about using too much; it's not going to hurt you at all, nor will it hurt the denture. This will help restore the suction and stability that you had before the denture broke. Obviously, you can buy the denture stickum at the pharmacy. I suggest using the paste instead of the powder. It seems to have more lasting power. Just squeeze a bunch on the individual fractured parts, place the segments back in your mouth and gently close down. You'll know when your bite is correct. Using this technique you should even be able to get through a number of meals without any real problems. Don't try peanut brittle. Do get to the dentist as soon as you can.

In the event that you don't have any of the denture adhesive around and you must go to the store to buy it, just place the two or three large broken parts of the denture in your mouth, close until your bite feels correct and then play like you've got a broken jaw that's wired together. That way at least you won't have to walk out of the house without your teeth. What else can you do? Not much. Literally, shut up and get to the stickum store or to the dentist. A two-piece break is much easier to cope with than three pieces.

If the denture has to be sent out to a lab for the repair, be prepared to be without the denture for about two or three hours. If there is a lab at the dental office, all the better. Then the repair should take no longer than about half an hour.

A word of advice. If you do use the stickum, dentists despise having to clean that junk out of the denture. When you get to the office, be nice and offer to clean it out yourself. Trust me, it will be appreciated.

If you are genuinely talented with your hands and I don't recommend this, even if you're a da Vinci, you could try to glue the parts together as I described for a broken tooth. If you should fail and improperly oppose the pieces and can't get them apart again, you've not only created a situation where you might not be able to use the denture, but you might just have sent your dentist on a nice vacation. You may have bought yourself a new denture.

In attempting this technique, use the smallest amount of glue possible so that if you make a mistake, you can snap the pieces apart. My advice: Don't try it. Use adhesive instead and trust your dentist to repair the break properly.

Ill-Fitting Dentures

Dentures that don't fit properly can leave you with decreased chewing ability, loose, clickety-clacking-like-train wheels-on-railroad-tracks teeth.

Poorly fitting dentures should be professionally relined. If for some reason, you can't have it done right away, here are a few basic ideas that will buy you some time. Yes, it's temporary treatment only, but it's inexpensive and effective.

Denture Pastes and Powders

Take your pick. There are many of these products on the market. Some people like pastes, some like powders. I happen to think that the pastes have a bit more holding power and are neater to use than are the powders. Squeeze some of the paste into the denture and reposition it in your mouth. Push firmly into place, using your thumbs for the upper and your index and middle fingers for the lower. Bite down, make sure that the bite is correct and that's that.

Make certain to keep your dentures exceptionally clean and change the stickum frequently, so as to prevent foul odors due to bacterial buildup. Let me tell you, the smell can be really nasty. Have you ever been in cattle country on a muggy day? That's roses in comparison. When removing the adhesive material for replacement, it will dissolve and wash out more readily in warm, rather than cold, water.

Whenever you are cleaning your dentures, do so over a sink that is partially filled with water. If the denture should fall, the water will prevent it from hitting the porcelain sink directly. It will soften the fall and minimize the possibility of the plate's breaking into a jigsaw puzzle.

Denture Pads

SeaBond is a brand name that comes to mind. No, I am not the president of the company, nor do I even know the president of the company. I happen to think it's a good product, not at all expensive, rather simple to use and quite effective in stabilizing loose dentures. Over the years I've told many of my patients with clacking dentures to purchase this product.

These adhesive pads (you get a number of them in a box) can be cut and formed easily. After trimming and moistening according to product instructions, place them inside the denture. They will fill in any voids between the denture base and the gums that may have been created by bone shrinkage. Because the pads have an adhesive embedded within their fibers, they will improve the stability and suction of your dentures, allowing you more confidence when talking and eating. The use of these pads can postpone the necessity of a reline for a reasonable period of time. What's reasonable? Who knows? Where economics plays an important role, you do what your pocketbook dictates.

Anyhow, the pads are quite soft and can also be exceptionally helpful in cushioning sore spots caused by poorly fitting dentures. You absolutely cannot damage your mouth or the dentures if these pads are used as directed. Try 'em, you'll like 'em!

Relines: What's and Why's?

There are few things more embarrassing than wearing dentures that seem to have a life and mind of their own. They can click out Morse code signals while you're talking or eating and perhaps give their impression of a flamenco dancer with castanets. They might even decide to go for a midnight swim in your sea of saliva.

As we age, we shrink, especially those parts of the body that no longer adequately function for their originally intended use. This holds true for the jawbone as well as other parts of the body. When teeth have to be extracted, the bone that held those teeth in place is no longer needed for that purpose; therefore, it shrinks. Even after the initial healing following extractions and even after dentures are placed, the bone continues to shrink. The rate of atrophy is very rapid at first, but is reduced drastically over the years. It does, however, continue throughout life.

Because of this ongoing deterioration, spaces are created between the dentures and the parts of the mouth on which they rest. It is for this precise reason that dentures made for you some years back will not fit as snugly as they did when originally fitted. The dentures become loose, wobbly and fit rather sloppily. When this happens, they must be relined.

The reline procedure is nothing more than the addition of more material to the pink denture base. This new material is very similar to that of the existing denture. It actually bonds to the plate, filling in any voids created by gum and bone shrinkage.

Some people require more relines over the years than others. This is because shrinkage occurs at different rates on different people. Relines might be necessary every year or so, depending on your age. Younger people may need more frequent relining than the elderly. Bone shrinkage is significantly reduced in the older generations.

A well-made denture, with relines done every few years, can serve you well for a long time. I hate to say it, but the most ideal reline can be accomplished only through the combined efforts of your ever-popular dentist and his lab technicians. When getting the denture relined, be prepared to be without it for at least four hours.

The technique, in case you're interested, is as follows:

1. The dentist smears a gooey material inside the denture, places it in your mouth and has you bite down for a couple of minutes. It'll seem like hours.

2. After the material sets, the denture is removed from your mouth and sent to the lab where the goo is removed. After plaster models are made, pink acrylic, very similar to your denture plastic, is placed into the denture and is heat cured to the denture base itself. This material fills in the voids between the denture and the gums that have been created over the years by bone shrinkage.

3. The denture is returned to the dental office. You come out of the closet and the denture is replaced in your mouth. That's that. You may have to return to the dentist for an adjustment or two, but that's a breeze.

Once, and as long as I live I will never forget this, I sent a denture out to the lab for a reline. The patient returned a couple of hours later to pick up the plate. The lab delivery hadn't arrived yet, so I had the patient come into my private office and wait and wait and wait. I became concerned and called the lab. They informed me that their delivery man had already left for my office some time ago. We tracked him down. He had been in an auto accident and was taken to the hospital emergency room for x-rays. He ended up with a broken arm. Fortunately, no one else was hurt. But where was the denture?

The owner of the lab returned to the scene of the accident. The car had been towed to a garage. He found the garage through the police report and got there as fast as he could. He opened the car door and there was the denture, in the back seat of the car, uninjured. No x-rays were necessary. Nothing was broken.

The denture was finally replaced in the patient's mouth at 9:00 p.m., some five hours after the patient returned to my office to pick up the case. If you think the patient breathed a sigh of relief, think about me. I had visions of shotguns running through my mind.

Home Reline Kits

Be careful. Although these materials are good and can last for months at a time, they are rather technique sensitive. You must follow the product instructions thoroughly. If used improperly, the denture can be badly damaged, sometimes beyond repair. Make certain that the brand you purchase states clearly that the material can be easily removed from your denture at a later time.

Don't forget, this material is only temporary and will start to disintegrate after a while, requiring replacement. If you routinely use these kits, clean out has to be done at regular intervals. As the material deteriorates, fungus growth can develop, which can be transmitted to your mouth tissues.

To clean out the mess, you must immerse your denture in hot water for about ten minutes. Then you have to try to peel the material from the denture. Be very cautious here. If the water is too hot, the hard plastic material of which the denture is made can soften and distort to the point that your denture might become a useless piece of plastic. You may not be able to wear it at all.

Again, when used correctly, this stuff is fantastic and relatively long lasting. Unfortunately, when it's used improperly your denture could be irreversibly damaged. It could prove to be a costly error.

Please don't be afraid to use this type of product. I'm not trying to scare you. I just want to impress you with the importance of following product instructions. If instructions are read and carefully obeyed, you can save bucks. If they are not, it's going to cost you.

Chapter 7: Other Dental and Mouth Issues

Bad Breath: The Gruesome Word, "Halitosis"

Have you ever awakened with a dry mouth that tastes kind of like a cross between steaming cow manure and rotten eggs? This is because your salivary flow is diminished while you sleep and bacteria have an opportunity to grow. If it tastes like that to you, can you imagine what it smells like to someone else? You'll really know who your true friends are when you exhale.

Halitosis

There are some simple things you can do to improve your breath. The first is to brush your teeth and tongue at least twice a day. Floss. Keep your mouth moist to wash away excess bacteria. And see your dentist regularly.

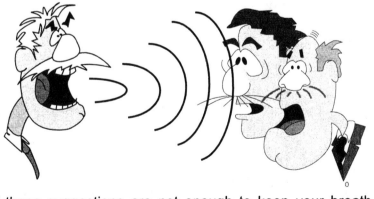

If these suggestions are not enough to keep your breath fresh, make an appointment with your family physician. Some other health problems may be involved.

Let's assume your bad breath is caused by "dry mouth," which simply means that there is a lack of saliva in your mouth. The saliva, in addition to helping you to swallow and start the digestive process, actually helps to mechanically wash away the gobs of bacteria that accumulate in the mouth. Lack of saliva allows the grubby bacteria to stay put, flourish, stink and create cavities.

Frequent brushing is extremely important to people with chronic dry mouth. Brushing is important, period. And guess what? Miracle of miracles, in addition to reducing the possibility of getting cavities, brushing also happens to minimize bad breath.

It all really boils down to a few basics. Follow a proper home oral-care program, which includes tooth *and* tongue brushing, flossing, using a Water Pik and keeping your mouth moist. See your dentist routinely. Breath sprays and mints are *not* forbidden fruit.

If bad breath truly can't be controlled by these simple methods and neither you nor your dentist can determine the cause, you should seriously consider seeing your family physician and having him check for other possible causes not originating directly from the mouth.

Treatment for bad breath can be extremely simple. Most everything is keyed into cleaning and moistening the mouth. Dry mouth and poor oral care, which both promote bacterial growth, are leading causes of bad breath. If the following treatments are properly and routinely followed, they can virtually eliminate those embarrassing moments when the world backs away from you rather rapidly each time you open your mouth and say h-h-h-e-e-e-l-l-l-o-o-o.

Brush your teeth properly. Bad breath can be caused by poor brushing habits. What an astonishing observation. Isn't that absolutely mind boggling?

Brush your teeth in an up and down motion, starting with the back teeth on one side, coming around to the front teeth and continuing to the back teeth on the other side. This should be done on both the cheek surfaces of the teeth as well as the surfaces that face the tongue. Finally, brush across the chewing surfaces. Proper brushing should take a good few minutes. If you have problems understanding my description of the brushing procedure, your dentist and his hygienist can instruct you in the proper techniques. This is one of those situations whereby a demonstration is worth a thousand words.

Routine use of baking soda is excellent as it helps reduce the bacterial count in the mouth. Dissolve a small amount in warm water placed in the "Water Pik." The Water what? I'll explain a little later on page 129.

Brush your tongue. Most people won't even consider tongue brushing to help keep the mouth clean. The top of the tongue is loaded with bacteria and dead tissue cells. This is also a major cause of bad breath. The tongue should be brushed along with the teeth, especially in the morning. A few gentle strokes from back to front will be sufficient. Stick your tongue out and start as far back on the tongue as is practical.

You don't have to brush back to your tonsils! Even if you were to brush from the midpoint forward, it would be beneficial.

I suggested this to a patient once. The patient had a very strong gag reflex and explained to me that the tongue brushing triggered this reflex, which caused her to throw up almost every time she tried to brush her tongue. This, of course, didn't do too much for the bad breath problem. After questioning her, I found that she was starting way too far back. She was brushing so far back that her toothbrush was touching that little dangling thing (uvula, for the trivia buffs) in the back of her mouth. Not necessary.

Try sucking on sugarless candies. They all tend to create saliva and some don't taste too bad either. Make certain that they are sugarless, because mixing sugar with the dry mouth syndrome is like putting a fox in the hen house. You're asking for trouble, just pleading for tooth decay.

Keep a bottle of water with you. Frequent sipping will obviously moisten the mouth and this is often all that is necessary to minimize, if not eliminate, bad breath associated with dry mouth. Don't gulp massive amounts. Sipping will do. Before swallowing, gently swish the water around in your mouth.

Chewing sugar free gum is excellent and tends to create copious amounts of saliva.

There are a number of commercial products available on the market that can be purchased without a prescription that will help to keep the mouth moist and help reduce bad breath. They usually come in a spray bottle and are advertised as "oral moisturizers" or "saliva substitutes." Personally, I like gum or sugarless candies. They taste better, they are cheaper and are more readily available.

Use mouthwashes, breath sprays and mints. These and other deodorants for the mouth are, for the most part, stopgap remedies, but I like them. They are temporary at best, lasting maybe ten to fifteen minutes. They're harmless and can be very effective for those "intimate moments," as long as they don't become "intimate hours." So, even though they are brief corrections, you won't be hurting anything by using them. I don't care which you use. Sprays, drops, mints, anything that helps. Besides, they taste good.

Mouthwashes containing zinc may be better than others because the zinc slows down the formation of sulfur compounds. Sulfur can promote bad breath. Read your labels.

Tooth decay must be corrected. Cavities mean rotten teeth. Rotten teeth stink. Get the cavities filled. Sorry, this book can't help you there.

Gum disease must be stopped. This goes hand in hand with lack of brushing and lack of proper professional care, as does the decay problem. Again, can't help you here. Gotta see the dentist. I do, however, give you some tips on gum problems beginning on page 69.

If you wear dentures, keep them spotlessly clean. Brush and care for them like they were your own teeth. There are special tooth pastes that will help keep them clean and fresh.

Quit smoking. Any questions about this one?

There are some conditions under which bad breath can actually be expected and should be considered as normal. We need not concern ourselves with these causes, other than to mention them, because for the most part they are self-correcting. They are as follows:

- after a recently extracted tooth,
- with a cold or sore throat,
- with a sinus infection, and
- after a good hearty meal loaded with garlic.

These causes are all essentially self-limiting.

Bad breath can also be caused by non-oral problems, such as stomach and lung disorders, as well as other systemic ailments. These are medical conditions that are not within the scope of this publication. Go see your physician.

Chapped Lips

This is ridiculously simple. Use any lip balm, Chapstick, etc., every hour or so. Try not to lick your lips as the moisture placed on the lips from the saliva will tend to dry rather quickly and will further aggravate the problem. When brushing your teeth, to prevent further irritation to the lips, use a non-flavored toothpaste. The flavoring might sting. Use baking powder if you like. Needless to say, stay away from spicy foods.

The lips don't have the same kind of oils that are contained in the rest of your face. Because of this, they will chap more readily and more severely. The dry, windy, winter months are the worst time for chapped lips. If the lips don't respond rapidly to treatment and the problem refuses to heal and if the corners of your mouth are always cracked and oozing, it's time to see the dentist or physician.

Jaw Joint Pain (TMJ Disorders)

The TMJ (temporomandibular joint) is the hinge joint, located directly in front of the ear. It allows the lower jaw to open and close and also move through its entire range of motion. The upper jaw, by the way, is not moveable. I'll bet that's something you never thought about. I'm certain that this fact will now remain in your conscious thoughts every moment of every day of your life.

Jaw (TMJ) Pain

The jaw has a hinge called the temporomandibular joint (TMJ) that lets you open and close your mouth. Injuries, poor bite, and even continually clenching your teeth can cause problems with this joint. Symptoms include severe headaches, neck stiffness, pain when eating, ringing in the ears and even hearing loss. If your jaw clicks and pops when you move it, you may have TMJ problems.

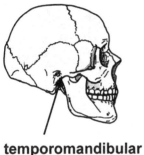

temporomandibular joint (TMJ)

Some of the things that help are gentle massage on the outside of the joint, heat, and pain relievers like aspirin or ibuprofen. Cold may also help to reduce sharp pain. Lowering your stress level so you don't clench your jaw as much may also bring long-term relief to chronic TMJ disorders. Surgery is not customarily recommended for chronic problems although it may be necessary in cases of severe injury.

There are many things that, over the years, can cause problems with this joint, ranging from trauma — due to a fall or a blow to the area — to such things as osteoarthritis or a poor bite, possibly caused by non-replacement of lost back teeth. Even the seemingly innocuous habit of continually clenching your teeth is one of the causes of this rather common and uncomfortable problem.

Symptoms can range from severe headaches and neck stiffness, to actual hearing loss, along with a constant ringing in the ears. Inability to open more than half to one inch is not uncommon. Moderate to severe pain when eating (especially when over-opening), is also a common symptom. Loud popping and/or clicking noises can often be heard not only by you, but by people nearby.

What you can do to relieve the pain depends somewhat on why your jaw is hurting. If you received some blow to the jaw, the problem will probably resolve itself in a week or two. Some of the ideas below will help ease the pain while you are waiting for the damaged tissue to heal.

A word of caution, if you received a blow and you have limited jaw motion, your teeth don't come together properly, or your jaw locks in an open position, you may have a fractured jaw and you should go to your dentist or the hospital emergency room.

For chronic pain, that is pain not related to a specific traumatic event, the treatment is usually just symptomatic, not curing the disease, *but treating the symptoms only.* Some ideas that work are listed below.

Gentle external massage over the joint area can help. This is usually the focal point of the pain. It's right in front of the ear. You can feel the joint easily when you open and close. Rub the area with your fingertips, using a gentle, circular motion, making certain not to clench your teeth when doing so. The massage will tend to relax the muscles overlying the joint.

Heat is excellent. Moist heat is better than dry heat, but if a hot, moist cloth is too messy and a hot water bottle isn't handy, a heating pad will do nicely. Heat will have a soothing effect on the jaw muscles. Find a comfortable chair, kick back and let the heat do its job. The heat is placed directly over the joint location, as was previously described.

Cold is also often a good treatment, especially if the pain is sharp, rather than just a dull ache. A frozen juice can or a bag of frozen vegetables wrapped in a towel makes a super cold compress. Ten to fifteen minutes on, followed by ten to fifteen minutes off is ideal. This sequence can be repeated a number of times throughout the day. If the ice pack is kept on too long and is not properly towel wrapped, you will come up with a severe case of frostbite, which helps absolutely nothing.

Your intelligent, deep-thinking author, with a degree in dentistry no less, left an ice pack on himself too long. The tissue turns black, sloughs off and takes a *very* long time to heal. Not a lot of fun and really hideous looking while it's healing. It happened to me only once. I learn fast.

Aspirin, as every one knows, is one of the miracle drugs of modern medicine. If there is no allergy or other medical reason not to take aspirin and the aspirin doesn't upset your stomach, it can be taken every four to six hours daily, as needed. It helps to reduce the inflammation in the joint, as well as minimize the pain involved. If you can't take aspirin, ibuprofen can also do an admirable job. Keep on the medication for about ten days to two weeks.

Don'ts (Simple, But Effective Suggestions)

- Don't over-open to eat that double quarter pounder with cheese.

- Don't open really wide when yawning, even if you're bored to tears.

- Don't eat crunchy, hard candies or tough, chewy foods. This includes gum, steaks (tender steaks are still wonderful), Abba Zabbas, Big Hunks, salt water taffy and all the other good things in life.

- Don't cradle the telephone between your shoulder and neck. This tends to put excessive pressure on the joint.

If there is no appreciable relief within two to four weeks, you should seriously consider seeing your physician or your dentist.

Most general practitioners, both dentists and physicians, will (or should) refer you to a specialist in the field. You must be extremely careful when accepting a referral. This is a highly specialized area and there are many professionals who envision themselves as being specialists when they are not. Do you get my drift?

If by any remote possibility, it is determined that surgery is necessary to alleviate the problem, make 1,000 per cent sure (that's one thousand, not one hundred) that your surgeon is well-experienced in the field, having many successful cases under his belt (or scalpel). A second opinion would be an excellent idea. You might consider having a staff member in the surgery department at a local dental school give you his or her input. Dental schools have excellent diagnosticians on staff and the fees are well below those that would normally be charged in private practice.

Please bear in mind that an unsuccessful surgery can leave you with even more severe problems than you had prior to surgery.

This surgery, as with any type of surgery, should be considered only when all else fails. Please pay attention! Did you get that? If not, read it again. Don't have surgery unless you absolutely have to. This is just common sense. If the discomfort is bearable, your surgeon may tell you to grin and bear it and treat the symptoms.

The success rate for this type surgery leaves much to be desired, regardless of the experience and expertise of the surgeon. Avoid, avoid, avoid, if at all possible.

Laryngitis Caused by Strain on the Vocal Cords

Although laryngitis, which is brought on by yelling too much at a sporting event and at your kids and even worse at your spouse, is not truly a dental problem, it's rather simple to handle.

- Suck on a mild, non-menthol, cough drop. This will tend to create moisture and help soothe your irritated throat. This should be done often throughout the day.

- Drown yourself with lots of water, sipping frequently. Sorry, no booze. Booze will ultimately dry the mouth and throat, as alcohol is a drying agent. The main thing is to keep the throat moist and shut up!

- Sipping old-fashioned tea and honey is very soothing. Oh yes, don't even consider talking above a whisper until that "strained" sensation in the throat is gone. Be calm and keep your blood pressure down to a low boil.

The laryngitis that I have just described is probably caused by the rupturing of small blood vessels in the throat. Yelling strains and ruptures these vessels. Talking above a whisper can slow down the healing. So again, s-s-h-h-h-u-t up and it'll go away in about three to five days. If not, see your doctor.

By the way, here's a situation where gargling with warm salt water is *not* a good idea. Those disgusting gurgling sounds made when you gargle can actually irritate, rather than help, your throat. Besides, I hate the taste of salt water.

Night Grinding (Also Known as Bruxism)

Symptoms and problems caused by grinding the teeth are varied, but the results are consistent with excess pressures being placed on the teeth and the jaws. Damage is being done. Some of the more common symptoms associated with grinding are sore jaws and teeth, loosened teeth, fractured teeth, wearing away of tooth structure, head and shoulder aches and, in the minds of many, the most important problem, keeping your spouse awake at night. The grinding can be genuinely noisy.

Night Grinding

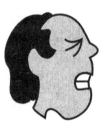

If you have a habit of clenching and grinding your teeth at night, you will probably wake up with sore jaws and teeth, worn teeth and complaints from your bed partner. (The last one may be the most immediate problem but the long-term damage will eventually hit you in the pocket book, too.)

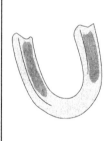

Your dentist can make you a bite plate to wear at night to keep your teeth from grinding on each other. You can actually make your own for a lot less money by using a football mouth guard. If that doesn't work, your dentist can make one with different materials that will probably work better.

Since the grinding is usually done routinely and unconsciously, it may be necessary for the dentist to make a soft plastic bite plate that fits over the teeth, to be worn while you sleep. This prevents the top and bottom teeth from contacting each other. The appliance actually serves as a shock absorber. It isn't a cure, but it will reduce soreness and minimize the damage that could otherwise be done to the teeth. The device can cost anywhere from $350 to $600, depending on your dentist's office overhead.

I've got a tip for you. If economics is a factor and you don't have a spare $600 hanging around, here's what to do:

Go into a sporting goods store and purchase a moldable football mouth guard. It will cost you about $5. Follow the product instructions carefully and you can make your own appliance. When making this bite plate, as you are contouring it to fit in your mouth, bite down into the soft plastic until your teeth are about 1/16 of an inch from contacting each other. Let it set in that position. This is usually a comfortable amount of opening and will prevent direct contact between your upper and lower teeth. Trim the edges to your liking. Wear it for a few nights while you sleep to see if it works. If your jaws and teeth are not sore in the morning, then it's doing the job. I'm assuming you have been awakening with sore jaws, because most everyone that night grinds, does.

If it doesn't work and the symptoms remain the same or get worse, we've failed and you're out five bucks, but it's still not a bad gamble. Then you'd best see the dentist to get a professionally made bite plate.

Night grinding is really a misnomer. It's generally done all day long as well as in the evening. Stress and tension are two major factors in causing this problem. Treatment of these underlying causes will not be addressed here as I am not qualified to hold stress management seminars.

Chapter 8: First Aid Kit and Other Supplies

Dental First Aid Kit

One of the simplest, yet one of the most frequently neglected, items that should be readily available to you in your home is a basic dental first aid kit. It would, as a matter of fact, be so easy to throw together that it could (and should) be placed into your shaving kit or makeup bag for travel purposes. Let's assume that you already have a medical kit available, so I won't mention general medications such as pain pills or antibiotics. I'll be as "dental specific" as possible.

Some of the items listed below will contain explicit manufacturer instructions. It is important that these directions be followed exactly, according to specifications, so that the product itself will function properly. In addition, there are instructions in this book located in the chapters relating to specific dental problems where these products would be useful. My instructions describe the technique for using the product in a dental situation and should be followed along with proper product handling. Please refer to those particular chapters.

The following is what I think would be necessary to complete a simple, compact dental first aid kit.

1. A piece of cotton. To be used if you have irritation from dentures or braces.

2. A teabag. To be used for control of bleeding after oral surgery.

3. Orabase or Orabase B, the mouth bandage.

4. Beeswax. To be used to cover sharp edges on orthodontic bands.

5. Temporary filling material. To be used if a filling falls out or breaks. This is superior to wax and worth getting for the kit.

6. Denture adhesive paste. Get a small sample tube from your dentist. To be used for a number of purposes:

   A. To make your denture more secure.

   B. To temporarily secure a cap or bridge that has come loose.

   C. To temporarily help stabilize a denture that has broken.

7. A packet of Stimudents. To help remove foreign objects that may have lodged between teeth.

8. Any brand of topical anesthetic that contains Benzocaine. Temporary relief for:

   A. Cold sores, fever blisters, canker sores.

   B. Denture sores.

   C. Any gum irritation.

   D. Have you ever bitten your lip, cheek or tongue? This'll help.

9. Toothache drops. Made from oil of cloves. When applied directly to the tooth with a cotton applicator, this can give some relief from moderate toothache pain.

10. A couple of packets of table salt from the local fast food restaurant. These will come in handy if rinsing is needed for any reason.

11. Gauze for wrapping a knocked-out tooth.

12. Clean cloth to use as a compress for cut cheeks, lips or gums. Black or red minimizes the amount of blood that you will see.

If you or someone in your family wears dentures or removable partial dentures, have a small separate kit available with the following items enclosed. Don't be concerned about duplication of products in the two kits. The cost is negligible.

1. A commercial denture cleaning powder (Efferdent, Polident).

2. A white candle as close to the color of your denture teeth as possible. A birthday candle is good. You can turn it into a fake tooth if one falls out.

3. Denture adhesive and/or denture pads.

4. A small bottle of rubbing alcohol. (See the section on denture repairs.)

5. Nail polish remover.

6. Super Glue or its equivalent. To be used in the following situations:

   A. To bind parts of broken denture base together. (*Please*, be very careful).

   B. To replace a denture tooth that may have popped off.

These products are all readily available at your pharmacy, but when you really want them they are nowhere to be found (at least not at home where they should be). Please go buy these things now and put them all somewhere in your bathroom. As I suggested, your travel kit, make-up kit or shaving kit is just fine. The items can be stored in a zipper type freezer bag. They'll all be *exactly* where you can find them when needed.

If you need one item in this kit, one time only, it will be worth far more to you in convenience than the minimal initial cost.

Toothbrushes and Toothpastes

Which do you think is more important, the paste that you use or the toothbrush? Without a doubt it's the brush and even more importantly, how it is used.

All toothpastes are essentially the same, being composed of an abrasive to help scrub the teeth, a flavoring to make it taste nice so that you'll purchase the same brand again and a binder to hold everything together. Oh yes, they do add fluoride and desensitizing agents, but we're talking basics, not bells and whistles.

The brush is the instrument that really does the cleaning of the teeth and the massaging of the gums. The operators of the brush, you and I, make the brush function properly or improperly.

I don't care if it's an electric brush, one with round bristles, one with flat bristles, one with an angled head, one with longer bristles on the outside and shorter ones on the inside. The important thing is to *have a brush and use it*. Replacement once every three months is sufficient. (A good way to remember when to replace your toothbrush is to get a new one the first day of each season, e.g., the first day of spring, the first day of summer and so on.)

Toothpaste is good to help control staining on the teeth due to its abrasive quality. It also gives a rather pleasant taste. Really, that's about it. Buy the least expensive, tastiest brand. As long as it is recommended by the ADA (American Dental Association), it's just fine.

Smoker's toothpastes are nothing more than pastes that contain a stronger, heavier abrasive. You can use them once in a while if your teeth tend to pick up a lot of staining from tobacco (quit, please), coffee or tea. Don't use them routinely. Don't let the kids use them at all.

One more thing. Don't be too vigorous about your brushing. Too much brushing with too much pressure can actually wear away tooth structure. Get a nice soft brush and be firm, but gentle. I've seen people who are so fanatic about brushing that it almost becomes a compulsive behavior.

This type of brushing can literally destroy tooth structure, especially near the gum line where the outer enamel is exceptionally thin. This can lead to exquisite sensitivity. Take it easy.

Water Pik

What is the Water Pik, you ask? Well, I'm going to tell you. I think it's one of the best dental hygiene instruments since the invention of the toothbrush.

The Water Pik is a fantastic appliance that no household should be without. It's a rather messy, but effective, aid to brushing and flossing that utilizes pulsating jets of water to help clean out crud that has accumulated between the teeth. It's also useful to squirt people from across the room.

Try this experiment: Do it at home, not at work.

Read product instructions completely and carefully. You *can* damage your mouth if you don't use it properly.

Brush your teeth thoroughly until you think your mouth is sparkling clean. Then go ahead and floss. When you feel that you have every little morsel of garbage cleaned out from between your teeth, use the Water Pik. You'll be amazed. Sometimes you'll get an entire meal out from between your teeth. Put it in the freezer, it'll be good for the budget. The Water Pik will clean out junk that you'd never imagine could get stuck in your mouth.

To repeat, consistent use of this appliance, regular dental checkups, along with brushing and flossing, can reduce the incidence of bad breath, as well as diminish the probability of developing cavities and gum disease.

Index

About the Author

I was born in New York way back in November 1936. My family migrated to California when I was seven. We all had a heavy Brooklyn accent (almost like foreigners). To this day people say I still have the remnants of that distinctive voice inflection. Can you hear it in my writing?

I went to grammar school and high school in Tujunga, California, a small town located in the San Fernando Valley just north of Los Angeles. This would ultimately be where I set up practice for thirty-five years.

I did my undergraduate work at the University of California in Berkeley during the "beatnik" years. (If you're old enough, you'll remember.)

I entered the University of California Dental School in San Francisco in 1956 and graduated four years later. I found school to be challenging, but rewarding. While in school my interests seemed to drift toward emergency care. I retained that interest throughout my years of practice. My claim to fame was that I, at age twenty-three, was the youngest graduating dentist in the United States.

Okinawa, with the United States Air Force, was my next stopping point. This gave me the opportunity to travel around the Orient, including Japan, Taiwan, Mainland China and Thailand. Visiting dental schools during my travels made me appreciate the Western methods of teaching dentistry. I also learned an awful lot about basic emergency dental procedures while in the service, something that was not really taught in school. After two years in Okinawa I returned to California and opened my private practice in early 1962.

Initially, when my office was first opened, I wasn't too busy. No one was knocking down the doors to see, or get drilled by, the "new kid on the block." I supplemented my income by helping to start one of the first hospital dental emergency facilities in the Los Angeles area. Unfortunately, the equipment was rather antiquated and the supplies were kept to a bare minimum.

The clinic, much to my displeasure, ultimately closed. To this day, twenty-four hour emergency facilities for dental care are few and far between. I suppose that "the powers that be" have never experienced a severe toothache.

I continued in my private practice, in the same building, until I finally called it quits in mid-1996. I stayed on with the new dentist for a period of months to make certain that the transition for him and the patients (and for me) was a smooth one. It wasn't. But that's another story.

I have been married now for 30 years. We have four children and four small grandchildren. My wife and I live with our youngest son in Valencia, California. Totally enjoying retirement, I really felt the need for a book of this nature. I wanted to inform the public of some simple, cost-effective ways to minimize the discomfort or inconveniences of certain problems associated with the mouth.

So I took precious time from my skiing and golf and went to work again, this time writing about dentistry rather than practicing. I am rather happy with the results and I hope that you will also feel the same.